MEMORY BANK FOR HEMODYNAMIC MONITORING

The Jones and Bartlett Pocket-Sized Nursing Reference Series

Chemotherapy Care Plans: Designs for Nursing Care
Barton Burke/Wilkes/Ingwersen

*Drugs and Protocols Common to Prehospital
and Emergency Care*
Cummings

*The EMS Pocket Drug Manual: A Quick Reference
Guide to Over 3,500 Drugs*
Dillman

1991-1992 Handbook of Intravenous Medications
Nentwich

Handbook of Oncology Nursing, Second Edition
Johnson/Gross

Memory Bank for Chemotherapy, Second Edition
Preston/Wilfinger

*Memory Bank for Critical Care: EKGs and
Cardiac Drugs, Third Edition*
Ervin

*Memory Bank for Hemodynamic Monitoring
The Pulmonary Artery Catheter, Second Edition*
Ervin/Long

*Memory Bank for Intravenous Therapy
Second Edition*
Weinstein

Memory Bank for Medications, Second Edition
Kostin/Sieloff

Oncology Nursing Drug Handbook
Wilkes/Ingwersen/Barton Burke

Ready Reference for Critical Care
Strawn/Stewart

MEMORY BANK FOR HEMODYNAMIC MONITORING

2nd Edition

The Pulmonary Artery Catheter

Gary W. Ervin, RN
Coronary Care Unit
Kaiser Foundation Hospital Medical Center
Hollywood, California

Sylvia Long, RN, BSN
Cardiac Intensive Care Unit
Cedars-Sinai Medical Center
Los Angeles, California

Jones and Bartlett Publishers
Boston   London

Library of Congress Cataloging-in-Publication Data

Ervin, Gary W., 1940-
    Memory bank for hemodynamic monitoring / Gary W. Ervin, Sylvia Long. - 2nd
ed.
        p. c   cm.
    Originally published: Baltimore: Williams & Wilkins, c1990.
    Includes bibliographical references.
    ISBN 0-86720-646-2
    1. Pulmonary artery-Catheterization-Handbooks, manuals, etc.
    2. Hemodynamic monitoring-Handbooks, manuals, etc.   I. Long,
Sylvia, 1939-   II.title
    [DNLM: 1. Heart Catheterization-instrumentation-handbooks.
    2. Heart Catheterization--instrumentation-nurses' instruction.
    3. Monitoring, Physiologic-handbooks.   4.   Monitoring, Physiologic-
-nurses' instruction.   WG 39   E72m 1990a]
    [RC683.5.P84E78   1993]
    616.1'20754-dc20
    DNLM/DLC   89-14660
    for Library of Congress   CIP

Printed in the United States of America
97 96 95 94 93   10 9 8 7 6 5 4 3 2

Preface

Routine electrocardiographic monitoring of critically ill patients preceded hemodynamic monitoring by about 10 years. It was not until the balloon-tipped, flow-directed pulmonary artery catheter was developed by H. J. C. Swan, MD, PhD, and William Ganz, MD, DSc, in the 1960s, that hemodynamic monitoring became commonplace in the critical care setting. This catheter not only made possible the bedside monitoring of hemodynamic parameters, it also made such monitoring practical.

As diagnostic techniques improve with technology, one fact remains constant. The validity of collected data depends upon accurate, consistent measurement and interpretation. The proper application of data provides both maximum usage and uniformity of results. **Memory Bank for Hemodynamic Monitoring, Second Edition,** has been developed to provide expert assistance in this vital area.

This book is a ready reference on management of hemodynamic monitoring with the pulmonary artery catheter. **Memory Bank for Hemodynamic Monitoring, Second Edition**, heightens comprehension, enhances retention, and facilitates application.

Special acknowledgment and appreciation for their assistance in the preparation and review of this manuscript are extended to Terri Forshee, RN, MSN, CCRN, and H. J. C. Swan, MD, PhD, Director, Division of Cardiology, Cedars-Sinai Medical Center, Professor of Medicine, UCLA School of Medicine, Los Angeles, California.

Gary W. Ervin
Sylvia Long

Figures and Tables

Figures

1.1   Swan-Ganz PA Catheter
      Showing Lumina and Ports . . .   2

1.2   Swan-Ganz PA Catheter with
      Balloon Inflated   4

1.3   Cross-Section of a Swan-Ganz
      Catheter with Thermodilution
      Wires   6

1.4   Heart in Diastole
      (Unichamber)   10

2.1   PA Catheter with Sterile
      Sleeve   21

2.2   Sterile Sleeve and Side Port
      IV Extension   22

2.3   Waveform Sequence   27

2.4   Normal Waveforms: Sequence,
      Shape, and Pressures Expected
      during Insertion   29

2.5   PA Catheter Positions and
      Corresponding Waveforms . .   30

2.6   Unlocked, Locked Balloon
      Lumen   34

2.7   Normal Cardiac Pressure
      Values   36

3.1   Zero Port Level with Zero
      Reference Point   49

5.1   Graph Paper with Scales . . .   74

5.2   PA Pressure Topping Out at
      Scale 40/10   75

5.3   PA Pressure in Figure 5.2
      read on a 200 Scale   76

5.4   EKG and PA Tracing at Speeds
      of 5, 10, and 25 mm/second,
      on a Scale of 40   80

5.5   PA Tracing with Respiratory
      Variation   82

5.6 Atrial Fibrillation: PA Pressures Vary with RV Stroke Volume ... 84
5.7 PAW with PEEP on a Mechanical Ventilator ... 86
5.8 Combining Scales, Scale 40/10 ... 88
5.9 Combining Scales, Scale 200/10 ... 89
5.10 Measuring PAW Waveform Components ... 92
5.11 Digital Readout Error ... 94
5.12 Cardiac Cycle: Heart Sounds, EKG, Waveforms, Valvular Motion ... 96
5.13 Right Atrial Waveform Components and EKG ... 100
5.14 Right Ventricular Waveform Components and EKG ... 102
5.15 Pulmonary Artery Waveform Components and EKG ... 104
5.16 Normal RA ... 106

5.17 Elevated RA ... 107
5.18 Extremely Elevated RA ... 108
5.19 Normal RV ... 109
5.20 Elevated RV ... 110
5.21 Progression of RA to RV ... 112
5.22 RV to PA ... 114
5.23 RV to PA, Balloon Inflated ... 116
5.24 RV Compared to PA ... 118
5.25 Elevated PA ... 120
5.26 Extremely Elevated PA ... 122
5.27 Normal PAW ... 124
5.28 PA to PAW: Elevated Pressures ... 125
5.29 Extremely Elevated PAW ... 126
5.30 Continuous Wedge ... 127
5.31 Overwedged Tracing ... 129
5.32 Catheter Whip/Fling ... 131
5.33 PAW Tracing ... 133
5.34 Equalized Pressures ... 134
5.35 PAW Tracing ... 136
5.36 PAW with V Waves ... 138
5.37 PAW Tracing ... 143

2.3 Approximate Insertion
       Distances 28

3.1 CDC Guidelines for the Preven-
       tion of Infections Related to In-
       travascular Pressure Monitoring
       Systems 53

4.1 Implications of Cardiac Index
       Readings 69

5.1 Implications of PAW
       Pressure 146

5.38 PA to PAW 144
5.39 RA Tracing 149
5.40 RA Tracing Suggesting
        Tricuspid Regurgitation 150

Tables
2.1 Insertion Sites and
       Techniques 15
2.2 Sizes 5 to 7.5 French PA
       Catheters 25

Contents

SECTION 1: The Pulmonary Artery Catheter 1

A. Description 2
B. Characteristics 3
C. Uses 7
D. Principles of PAW Measurement 11

SECTION 2: Insertion of the Pulmonary Artery Catheter 13

A. Preparation 14
  1. Nursing Responsibilities 14
  2. Equipment and Supplies 15
    a. Emergency Equipment 15
    b. Monitor/Flush System 16
    c. Skin Prep Supplies 16
    d. Setup Materials 17
    e. PA Catheter and Sterile Supplies 17
  3. Sterile Setup and Skin Prep Procedure 20
B. **Insertion** **23**
  1. Procedure 24
  2. Nursing Responsibilities *during* Insertion 28
  3. Points to Remember during Insertion 31
C. **Potential Complications during Insertion** **37**
  1. Dysrhythmias 37
  2. Kinking or Knotting of the Catheter .. 38
  3. Right Ventricle Perforation 39
  4. Pulmonary Artery Perforation 40
  5. Air Embolism 41

6. Bradycardia: Right Bundle Branch
   Block, Left Bundle Branch Block, or
   Complete Heart Block 42
7. Supraventricular Tachycardia 43
8. Pneumothorax 44
9. Venospasm 45

**SECTION 3: Care of the Patient with an
Indwelling PA Catheter** **47**

A. Nursing Responsibilities **48**
B. Potential Complications
   Postinsertion **52**
   1. Infection 52
   2. Displacement of Catheter 54
   3. Hemorrhage 55
   4. Pulmonary Thromboembolism 56
   5. Air Embolism 57
   6. Pneumothorax 57

**SECTION 4: Measurement of Cardiac
Output** **59**

A. Cardiac Output (CO) **60**
   1. Definition 60
   2. Uses 60
   3. Three Factors Affecting Stroke
      Volume 61
   4. Cardiac Index (CI) 62
B. Causes of *Low* Cardiac Output **63**
C. Causes of *High* Cardiac Output **63**
D. Treatment to Increase Cardiac
   Output **64**
E. Computing Cardiac Output by
   Thermodilution **64**
   1. Principle 64
   2. Points to Remember 65
   3. Supplies 67
   4. Procedure 68
F. Causes of Error in Cardiac Output
   Measurement **70**

Contents   **xiii**

SECTION 5: Waveforms and Pressures **71**

A. Scales and Speeds **72**
  1. Pressure Values 72
  2. Graph Paper 73
  3. Pressure Scales 73
  4. Monitor Scales 77
  5. Paper Speed 78
B. Pressure Complexes **79**
  1. Measurement 79
  2. Combining Scales 83
  3. Measuring Waveform Components .. 90
  4. Digital Readout Errors 91
C. Waveforms and Components **91**
  1. Right Atrial Waveform 98
  2. Right Ventricular Waveform......... 98
  3. Pulmonary Artery Waveform 99
D. Pressure Tracings **106**
  1. Right Atrial 106
  2. Right Ventricular 109

  3. Pulmonary Artery 118
  4. Pulmonary Artery Wedge 124
E. Diagnostic Pressures **132**
  1. Congestive Heart Failure 132
  2. Cardiac Tamponade 137
  3. Hypovolemia 137
  4. Mitral Valve Regurgitation 140
  5. Mitral Valve Stenosis 141
  6. Pulmonary Edema 142
  7. Pulmonary Embolus 146
  8. Pulmonary Hypertension 147
  9. Right Ventricular Infarct 147
  10. Septic Shock 148
  11. Tricuspid Valve Regurgitation 148
  12. Tricuspid Valve Stenosis 152

Appendix 1 Maintenance of Line
                Integrity 153
Appendix 2 Troubleshooting the PA
                Catheter 168
Appendix 3 Maneuvers to Eradicate
                Line Damping 169

Appendix 4 Infection Prevention and
Control 170

Appendix 5 Cardiac Therapy Indicated
by Subsets of Hemo-
dynamic Parameters... 176

Appendix 6 Definitions 180

Appendix 7 Commonly Used Vasoactive Drugs and
Nomograms 190

Appendix 8 Formulas 201

Appendix 9 Blood Gases 206

Appendix 10 Hemodynamic
Parameters 208

Appendix 11 BSA Chart 210

Appendix 12 Abbreviations........ 212

Bibliography 213

SECTION 1

The Pulmonary Artery Catheter

A. Description

A flexible, balloon-tipped, flow-directed catheter containing two to five inner lumens, for selected hemodynamic assessment, monitoring, and therapeutic purposes. The number of lumens depends on which hemodynamic parameters are to be measured.

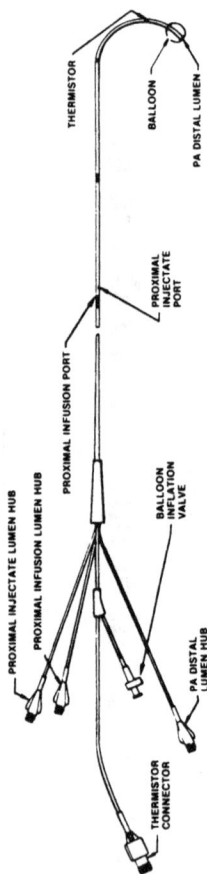

Courtesy of Edwards Labs.

Figure 1.1   Swan-Ganz PA Catheter Showing Lumens and Ports.

B. Characteristics

1. Made of polyvinyl chloride, which provides flexibility; is radiopaque, thus allowing for visualization of placement within the pulmonary artery.

2. Sizes 5, 6, 7, or 7.5 French. Total length is 110 cm; increments are marked at 10-cm intervals along the outer surface.

3. Contains two to five lumina; each serves a specific purpose in assessment of cardiac function.

   a. The *distal lumen* opens at the tip of the catheter and measures pulmonary artery (PA) and pulmonary artery wedge (PAW) pressures.

   b. The *balloon lumen* ends about 1 cm proximal to the distal lumen. The balloon is made of thin latex; it surrounds, but does not cover, the catheter tip. As the catheter is advanced, the inflated balloon allows it to flow in a forward direction.

   c. The *thermistor lumen* terminates at a thermosensitive bead on the surface of the catheter about 4 cm from the distal tip. It contains

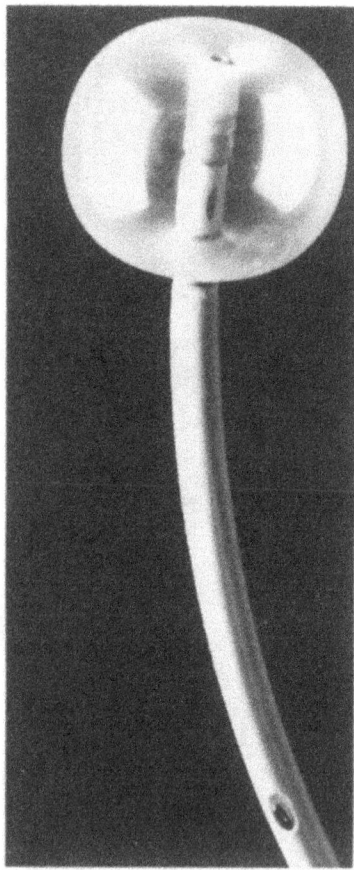

Courtesy of Edwards Labs.

Figure 1.2   Swan-Ganz PA Catheter with Balloon Inflated.

two, fine, insulated wires used to measure cardiac output using the thermodilution method.

d. The *proximal lumen* opens approximately 30 cm from the distal tip and is used to measure right atrial (RA) pressure and/or to infuse solutions. Some catheters contain two openings into the right atrium for simultaneous measurement and infusion.

e. Some catheters also incorporate pacing wires that can be connected to pacing electrodes and a pacemaker.

4. Each lumen has an entry port (figure 1.1).

a. The *distal lumen/PA port* connects via pressure tubing to a transducer, by which PA systolic, diastolic, and PAW pressures can be measured. Mixed venous blood samples are withdrawn from this lumen.

b. The *balloon lumen/balloon port* connects to a syringe for inflating air into the balloon and can be locked closed.

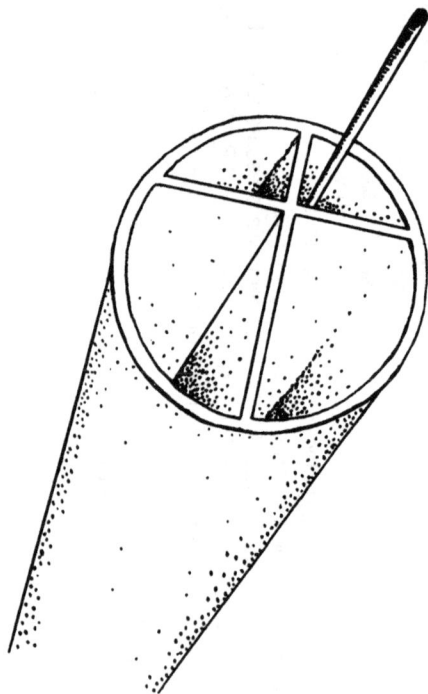

Figure 1.3   Cross-Section of a Swan-Ganz Catheter with Thermodilution Wires

c. The *thermister lumen/coupling port* connects the thermistor wires to a portable, bedside computer and is used to measure cardiac output and blood temperature.

d. The *proximal lumen/RA port* connects via pressure tubing to a transducer to measure central venous pressure (CVP). Injectates to measure cardiac output are instilled through this port. It also can serve as a line for IV infusions.

C. Uses

1. Pre-, intra-, and postoperative uses to
   a. Monitor high-risk patients[a]
   b. Monitor and treat high or low cardiac output states
   c. Monitor the patient when hypotensive anesthesia is used
   d. Monitor the elderly patient

---

[a]Patients with history of pulmonary/cardiac disease, angina, and potential fluid shifts during major surgery.

2. To assess, diagnose, and evaluate the effects of therapy in a variety of cardiopulmonary problems including
   a. Acute myocardial infarction
   b. Severe angina
   c. Congestive heart failure
   d. Cardiomyopathy
   e. Cardiac tamponade
   f. Pulmonary disease
   g. Right ventricular failure
   h. Intraoperative cardiac collapse

3. Specific monitoring to
   a. Differentiate cardiogenic from hypovolemic shock and evaluate the effect of therapeutic interventions
   b. Evaluate therapy in patients having severe and/or chronic heart failure with low cardiac output
   c. Evaluate therapy in patients having myocardial ischemia

d. Diagnose mitral regurgitation, ventricular septal rupture, or right ventricular infarction

e. Monitor cardiac function during use of parenteral vasoactive, inotropic, chronotropic, or diuretic agents used as preload and afterload therapy

f. Monitor cardiac function during use of intraaortic counterpulsation

4. Others

a. To diagnose pulmonary embolism

b. To monitor fluid balance, especially in patients with extensive trauma or burns, or who are elderly

c. As a research tool for clinical investigation

d. To obtain atrial electrocardiograms and/or initiate atrial pacing

Note: Contraindications for use may include patients with sepsis, a hypercoagulable state, or a left bundle branch block (unless a temporary pacing wire has been inserted).

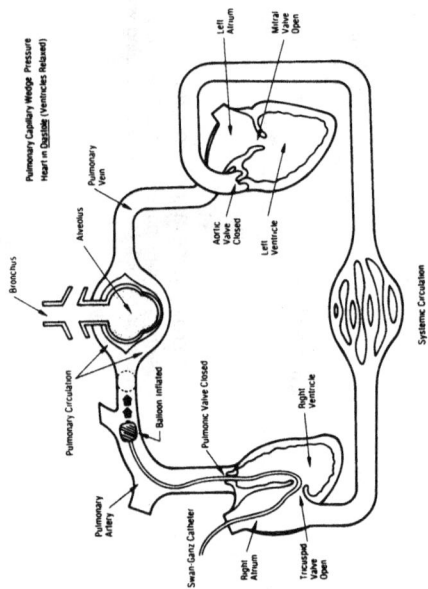

Courtesy of *Edwards Labs.*

Figure 1.4   Heart in Diastole (Unichamber)

D. Principles of PAW Measurement

1. After insertion, the pulmonary artery catheter lies in the main pulmo-nary artery or a primary branch. When the balloon is *not inflated*, the catheter measures pulmonary artery systolic and diastolic pressure. When the balloon *is inflated*, the catheter "floats" out to a smaller branch of the pulmonary artery, occludes it gently, and measures the pressure in front of the balloon; that is, pulmonary artery wedge (PAW) pressure.

2. During ventricular diastole, the mitral valve is open and the pressures in the left atrium and left ventricle equilibrate (figure 1.4). In the absence of mitral valve disease, mean PAW is closely approximate to the pressure in the left ventricle during diastole (LVDP): mean PAW = mean LVDP.

3. The LVDP roughly relates to ventricular volume in an individual patient. This pressure, as reflected by the PAW, indicates the earliest changes in the filling and function of the left ventricle.

SECTION 2

Insertion of the Pulmonary Artery Catheter

A. Preparation

1. Nursing Responsibilities

a. Obtain a signed consent after the MD has explained the procedure and risks to the patient.

b. Assemble and prepare the supplies and equipment.

c. Calibrate the transducer per manufacturer's directions.

d. Place the patient in the proper position with O_2 on (usual position is supine or Trendelenburg for a subclavian or Trendelenburg for a subclavian or internal jugular venipuncture; per patient's comfort for a peripheral insertion).

e. Connect patient to monitor and obtain a clear EKG tracing.

f. Obtain baseline vital signs.

g. Assist physician in gowning, drawing up solutions.

Table 2.1 Insertion Sites and Techniques

Site	Technique
Antecubital fossa vein	Cutdown
External or internal jugular vein	Percutaneous
Femoral vein	Percutaneous
Subclavian vein	Percutaneous

2. **Equipment and Supplies**[a]
   a. Emergency Equipment
      1) crash cart with defibrillator, pacemaker equipment, and advanced life support drugs

[a]Items will vary among hospitals.

2) O$_2$ setup

3) suction set with standard and tonsil tip catheters

4) EKG monitor

5) chest tube and water-seal suction

b. Monitor/Flush System

   1) pressure bag

   2) fluid transfer pack

   3) flush solutions

      a) cardiac patients: 5% D/W 500 ml with heparin 500 units

      b) other patients: normal saline 500 ml with heparin 500 units[b]

   4) IV tubing with macrodrip chamber

c. Skin Prep Supplies

   1) razor

   2) sterile towels

   3) sterile gloves

---

[b]Amount of heparin depends on hospital protocol.

4) 4 × 4s

5) forceps

6) Betadine Solution and Betadine Scrub[c] (for patients sensitive to iodine, Hibiclens is a good alternative)

d. Setup Materials

1) arm board (if peripheral site is anticipated)

2) soft wrist restraints, as necessary

3) caps and masks

4) hand scrub setup

5) sterile gown, gloves

6) transducer/manifold: calibrated, leveled, and air-zeroed

e. PA Catheter and Sterile Supplies

1) suture material

a) silk 3-0 and 4-0

b) chromic 4-0

[c]Solutions may vary among hospitals.

2) sterile umbilical tape

3) 3 sterile 5 or 10 ml syringes (for flushing proximal and distal lumina)

4) 1 sterile Tbc or 3 ml syringe (to inflate balloon; see table 2.2)

5) Xylocaine 1% or 2% (without epinephrine)

   a) 1 sterile 10 ml syringe

   b) 1 sterile 18 gauge needle

   c) 1 sterile 25 gauge needle

6) 3 sterile 3-way stopcocks

7) 1 scalpel handle with a #11 blade

8) 1 scissors and needle holder

9) 6 each sterile towels and towel clips

10) 1 small sterile bowl

11) pulmonary artery catheter, introducer, catheter guard shield, wire guide

12) 2 pressure tubings (4 feet) with male to male couplings

13) flush solution (pour 500 ml of 5% D/W or normal saline into sterile basin; add heparin[d] 500 units to make a concentration of 1 unit/ml)

14) if the insertion is to be percutaneous, add a #18 Cook, a #16 Cournand-Potts, or a #16 angiocath; a protective sterile sleeve (figure 2.1) may be slipped over the catheter; a side port extension (figure 2.2) may also be added to provide an additional IV line

15) if insertion is by cutdown, omit sterile supplies listed previously and add cutdown tray

---

[d]Amount of heparin depends on hospital protocol.

3. Sterile Setup and Skin Prep Procedure

ALERT PREPARATION FOR INSERTION OF THE PULMONARY ARTERY CATHETER REQUIRES STRICT ASEPTIC TECHNIQUE.

a. Setup: after assembling the equipment and supplies, open two sterile towels (or the cutdown tray) on a table or stand that can be placed over the bed or immediately beside the physician. Add sterile supplies (as listed, or per hospital protocol) and flush solution.

b. Skin Prep Procedure

1) ascertain specific site of insertion and shave area, if necessary

2) pour Betadine Scrub and Betadine Solution into two sterile containers

3) drop sterile 4 × 4s into containers of Betadine

4) put on sterile gloves, then drape site

5) scrub skin holding 4 × 4s in forceps

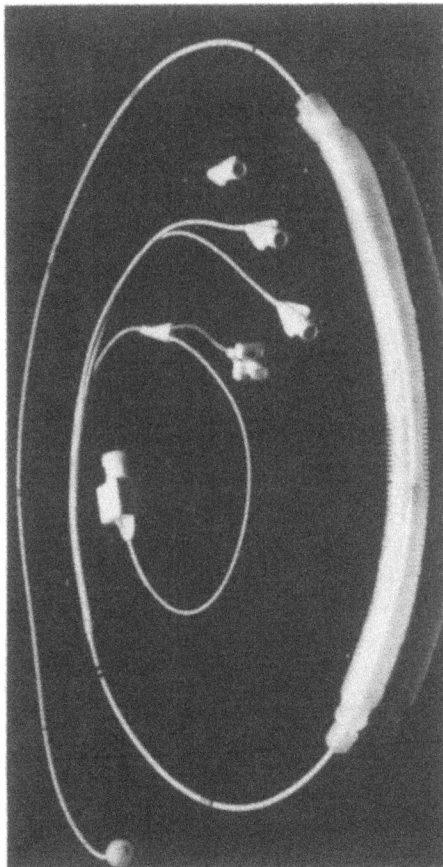

Courtesy of Edwards Labs.

Figure 2.1   PA Catheter with Sterile Sleeve

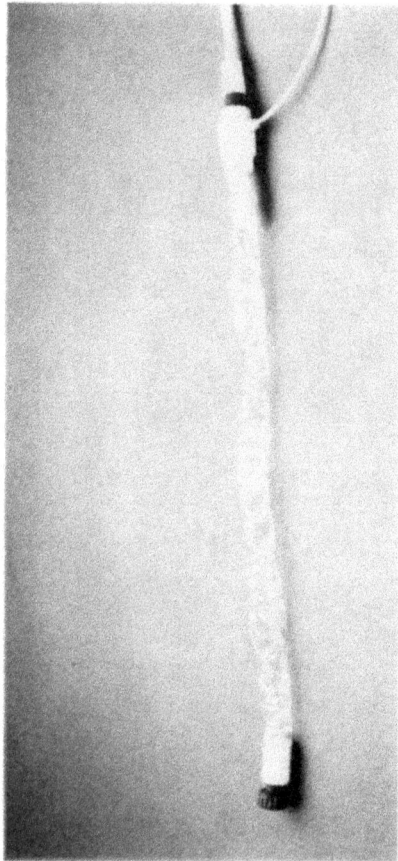

Courtesy of Argon Medical Corp.

Figure 2.2   Side Port IV Extension

a) use Betadine Scrub first, follow with Betadine Solution

b) beginning at the center of the site, scrub in a circular motion away from the center, using light friction

c) do *not* go back over the area with the same 4 × 4

d) discard used 4 × 4 into a receptacle below the clean area

e) with the forceps, select new 4 × 4s and repeat procedure for 5 minutes

6) cover the area with a sterile towel until the insertion precedure begins

B. Insertion

Note: This procedure must be performed by a physician only.

ALERT METICULOUS STERILE TECHNIQUE IS OF UTMOST IMPORTANCE

1. Procedure

a. Test the intactness of the balloon as follows:

1) connect syringe to the balloon port; inject air (table 2.2) while the catheter tip is submerged in sterile normal saline

2) if air bubbles appear from the balloon, it is not intact and another catheter must be selected

3) if the balloon is intact, check to see that (while inflated) it surrounds but does not occlude the catheter tip; if it covers the tip, replace and test as above

4) if the balloon is intact and surrounds the catheter tip, disconnect the syringe to allow passive deflation

5) expel all air from the syringe and connect it once again to the balloon port after the balloon has deflated (some prefer to keep syringe disconnected from balloon port to ensure against accidental or prolonged balloon inflation)

Table 2.2 Sizes 5 to 7.5 French PA Catheters

Size	# of Lumina	Maximum Balloon Volume	Suggested Syringe to Use
5 Fr	2	0.8	Tbc
6 Fr	3	1.5	3 ml
7 Fr	4 or 5	1.5	3 ml
7.5 Fr	5	1.5	3 ml

ALERT *NEVER INJECT FLUID INTO THE BALLOON.*

b. Flush the proximal and distal catheter lumina with heparinized solution to preclude air emboli. Wipe the outside of the catheter with
sterile 5% D/W or normal saline, and leave it moist (to reduce catheter surface tension).

c. Using either cutdown or percutaneous stick, insert a wire guide and venous introducer sheath into the vein. Remove the guide and thread the PA catheter through the sheath until the tip is near the junction of the vena cavae and the right atrium. Connect catheter to pressure tubing. Ask the patient to cough; if the catheter tip is in the thorax, this will result in a pressure of 40 mm Hg.

d. Inflate the balloon with air or CO_2. This will allow the catheter to flow in a forward direction as the catheter is advanced.

e. The catheter can now be advanced *carefully* (the waveforms will indicate when the right atrium is entered; see figure 2.3).

   1) monitor pulmonary artery pressure and EKG continuously

   2) if catheter has not wedged by the distance indicated in table 2.3, it may be coiled; if so, withdraw to RA and readvance

f. When the waveform is wedged, deflate the balloon and carefully advance 2 to 3 cm to compensate for recoil. While holding catheter in place, slowly inflate the balloon to check this position. Note the

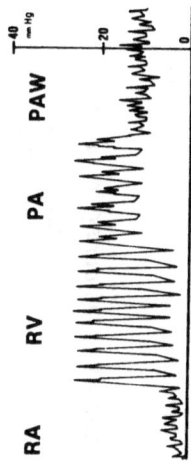

RA   RV   PA   PAW

Courtesy of Edward's Labs.

Figure 2.3   Waveform Sequence

volume of air required to inflate the balloon for a wedge waveform and record.

g. Note approximate length of insertion (in cm on catheter shaft) in case the catheter is pulled out or manipulated later. Anchor the catheter with sutures and tape it in the chevron style at the insertion site. Tape catheter securely to the hub of the introducer, since the two can disconnect and the catheter can inadvertently slip out of

Table 2.3   Approximate Insertion Distances

To junction of SVC and RA from:

Right antecubital fossa	= 40 cm
Left antecubital fossa	= 50 cm
External jugular vein	= 20 cm
Femoral vein	= 30 cm

Note: PAW should be obtained by advancing the catheter another 10 to 20 cm, depending upon the heart size.

the heart. Cleanse area with Betadine Solution, apply Betadine Ointment, and cover with an occlusive dressing.

h. Order an overpenetrated chest x-ray to check the position of the catheter.

2. Nursing Responsibilities *during* Insertion

a. Observe the patient for anxiety, level of consciousness, adequacy of ventilation, and pain. Maintain verbal and physical contact for

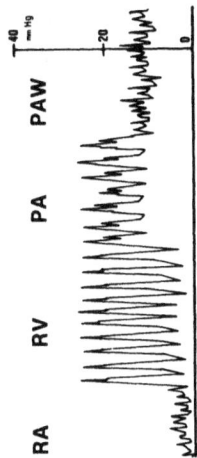

Courtesy of Edwards Labs.

Note: In disease states, the appearance and value of the waveforms will deviate from normal.

Figure 2.4 Sequence of Normal Waveforms and Pressures Expected During Insertion

RA: low undulating, 2–6 mm Hg
RV: rectangular, 25/2–25/6 mm Hg
PA: triangular 25/8–25/12 mm Hg
PAW: low W shape, 8–12 mm Hg

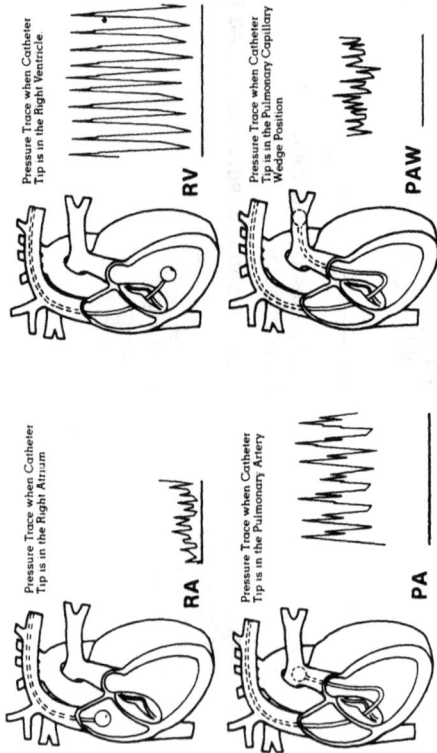

Pressure Trace when Catheter
Tip is in the Right Atrium

RA

Pressure Trace when Catheter
Tip is in the Right Ventricle

RV

Pressure Trace when Catheter
Tip is in the Pulmonary Artery

PA

Pressure Trace when Catheter
Tip is in the Pulmonary Capillary
Wedge Position

PAW

Courtesy of Edwards Labs.

Figure 2.5   PA Catheter Positions and Corresponding Waveforms

continuing reassurance and cooperation; provide as much information about procedure as patient wants.

b. Monitor vital signs at least every 15 minutes.

c. Observe EKG monitor for dysrhythmias; identify any and obtain a
printout. (Lidocaine may be necessary for prolonged V Tach or multiple PVCs.

d. Connect the catheter to fluid-flushed pressure tubing as directed by
physician.

e. Observe changing waveforms on oscilloscope as physician inserts
catheter (figure 2.4). Identify and record RA, RV, PA, and PAW tracings.

f. Measure cardiac output (see Chapter 4).

3. Points to Remember *during* Insertion

a. Watch waveforms and pressures to determine location of catheter
tip (figure 2.5); note any ventricular irritability induced by catheter
manipulation.

b. If difficulty in passing the catheter is encountered, injecting iced normal saline through the catheter may help by stiffening it.

c. If a PA or PAW pressure is not obtained after passing the catheter tip through the right ventricle, deflate the balloon and pull the catheter back to the right atrium (watch for RA pressure). Reinflate the balloon and advance again (to be done by physician only).

d. Patients with enlargement of the right atrium or right ventricle or with tricuspid incompetence are sometimes difficult to catheterize. In such cases the physician may try the following:

1) use a #7 Fr catheter with a *preshaped tip*; this catheter is somewhat stiffer than the #5 Fr, and the design of the tip aids advancement through the right heart.

2) ask the patient to inspire deeply while the catheter is being advanced (sometimes helps to obtain wedge by decreasing intrathoracic pressure and enhancing blood flow)

e. Once the balloon becomes wedged, deflate it. Never leave the balloon inflated for more than 15 *seconds* or two to three respiratory cycles in *any* patient, and especially not in an elderly patient or a patient with pulmonary hypertension. The best practice is to wedge the balloon, take the PAW reading, and immediately deflate it. Be careful *not* to lock the balloon in wedge (figure 2.6). (Many MDs/RNs prefer to disconnect the syringe from the balloon port when not taking a PAW pressure.)

ALERT A BALLOON LEFT IN WEDGE POSITION WILL CAUSE A PULMONARY INFARCTION

f. After the balloon is deflated, the catheter tip may recoil (backward displacement). At times, it may recoil back into the right ventricle and precipitate dysrhythmias. If this should happen, inflate the balloon and advance the catheter an additional 2 to 3 cm.[e]

---

[e]MD does this; RN can do if covered by written hospital protocol.

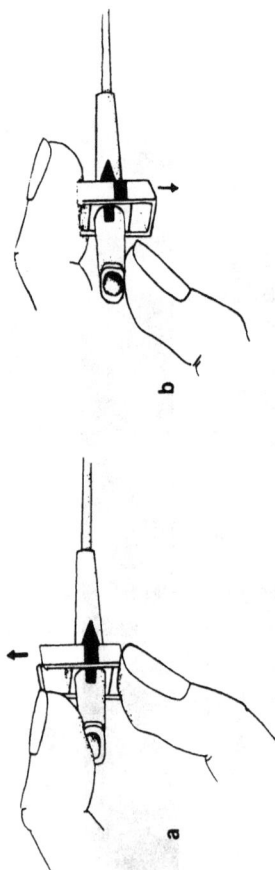

Figure 2.6   Unlocked (a), Locked (b) Balloon Lumen

g. The catheter may wedge spontaneously (forward displacement). Therefore, monitor pressures and waveforms constantly. When a continuous wedge is suspected, there is imminent danger of infarcting that portion of the vascular tree, and the catheter must be repositioned. Have the patient turn, cough, or (if an antecubital insertion) extend arm out perpendicular to body. If this is not successful, pull the catheter back 3 to 4 cm. *DO NOT* inflate the balloon or hand flush the PA lumen. Be sure that you are monitoring PA; RA can look like PAW, as can PA read on a 300 scale.

ALERT IF A CONTINUOUS WEDGE IS SUSPECTED, DO NOT INJECT FLUID THROUGH THE DISTAL PORT

h. To test for accuracy of catheter placement, inflate the balloon *very slowly* while watching the monitor. Once the pressure changes from

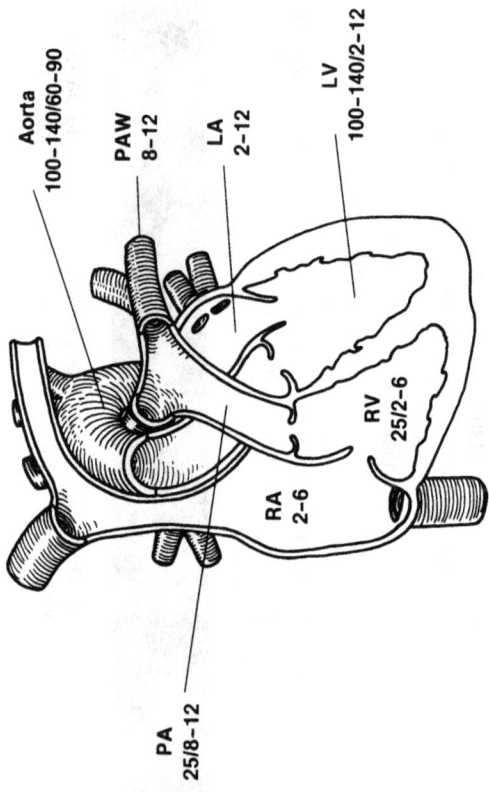

Aorta
100–140/60–90

PAW
8–12

LA
2–12

LV
100–140/2–12

RV
25/2–6

RA
2–6

PA
25/8–12

Figure 2.7 Normal Cardiac Pressure Values (Pressures are in mm Hg)

PA to PAW, do not inflate any further. If the volume of air or CO_2 that wedges the catheter is significantly below what is indicated on the catheter shaft or what initially wedged the catheter, the tip of the catheter may have migrated too far into the branch of the pulmonary artery; if so, pull the catheter back 2 to 3 cm.[f] Inflating the balloon to the 0.8 ml level in this instance could cause damage to this portion of the pulmonary artery.

C. Potential Complications during Insertion

1. Dysrhythmias (primarily PVCs, ventricular tachycardia, bradydysrhythmias, complete heart block)

Causes

a. Irritation of the endocardium by the catheter tip

b. Looping of excess catheter

---

[f]MD does this, RN can do if covered by written hospital protocol.

c. Recoil of the catheter tip from the PA back into the RV

Actions

a. Inflate the balloon.
b. Notify MD to reposition the catheter.
c. Give Lidocaine for sustained dysrhythmias (per hospital policy).
d. Withdraw catheter to RA.[g]

2. Kinking or Knotting of the Catheter[h]

Causes

a. Small, flexible catheter was used.
b. Excessive length was inserted (RV is normally reached 15 cm after RV).

---

[g]MD does this; RN can do if covered by written hospital protocol.
[h]Detected during fluoroscopy and by absence of waveforms.

Actions

a. Do not advance further if the RV or PA is not reached by the appropriate length (see table 2.3).

b. Notify MD, who will pull back excess catheter (for kinks) or untie knot under fluoroscopy.

3. Right Ventricle Perforation

Symptoms

a. Cardiac tamponade

b. Shock

c. Arrest

Cause

Recent RV infarct caused scar tissue and/or weakened area in RV wall.

ALERT THIS IS AN EMERGENCY

Actions

a. Notify surgeon STAT (surgical repair).
b. CPR if indicated.
c. Assemble equipment for pericardiocentesis.

4. Pulmonary Artery Perforation

Symptoms

a. Hemoptysis
b. Severe respiratory distress
c. Shock

Causes

a. Erosion by impacted catheter tip
b. Balloon inflation in small branch vessel

Actions

a. Notify physician STAT (depending on the patient's clinical status, surgical repair may be necessary).

b. CPR if indicated.

Note: Symptoms of PA perforation must be differentiated from those of severe pulmonary edema via clinical assessment and chest x-ray, and treated accordingly.

5. Air Embolism

Cause

Balloon rupture in the patient with a septal defect (intracardiac shunt); air enters the left ventricle and/or the aorta, causing a free air embolus.

Action

Position patient on left side with head lower than feet.

Prevention

Use CO_2 instead of air for inflating the balloon when shunting is suspected.

6. Bradycardia: Right Bundle Branch Block, Left Bundle Branch Block, or Complete Heart Block

Cause

The catheter mechanically damages the functional right bundle branch in a patient with left bundle branch block (LBBB).

ALERT THIS IS AN EMERGENCY

Actions

a. Withdraw catheter.
b. Emergency pacemaker
c. CPR as indicated

Prevention

Insert a temporary transvenous pacemaker in LBBB patients prior to inserting the pulmonary artery catheter.

7. Supraventricular Tachycardia

Causes

Wolff-Parkinson-White syndrome or Ebstein's anomaly

Actions

Give Verapamil or Pronestyl, as ordered.

Prevention

Sedate anxious patient prior to procedure. Diagnostic 12-lead EKG.

8. Pneumothorax

Cause

The apex of the thorax is pierced with the introducing needle during a subclavian insertion. This is more common in the restless patient or when insertion is done on left side of thorax.

Actions

a. Maintain verbal contact and provide as much information as patient wants, in order to decrease anxiety.

b. Instruct patient to take shallow rather than deep breaths.

c. Insert chest tube, connect to water-seal suction; and administer supplemental O_2.

Prevention

If the patient is restless, sedate prior to the procedure.

9. Venospasm

Cause
Irritation of the vessel during insertion

Actions
a. Pull catheter back 10-20 cm and briskly move it back and forth in 5 cm strokes.

b. Inject small amount of Lidocaine through distal port.

c. Apply heat to extremity for 15 minutes.

d. Use a smaller catheter.

ALERT DISCONTINUE INSERTION UNTIL VENOSPASM BREAKS

Continuing insertion during venospasm can lead to pain, vagal reaction, and hypotension.

SECTION 3

Care of the Patient with an Indwelling PA Catheter

A. Nursing Responsibilities

1. Monitor pressures and waveforms (PAW, PA, RA) constantly; record hourly and/or prn.

2. Flush lines hourly and prn (if automatic flushing devices are not being used).

3. Calibrate transducer with mercury every 8 hours; check air zero and calibration factors every 4 hours and prn.

4. Keep the transducer air-zero port level with the phlebostatic axis (right atrium) during pressure readings (figure 3.1). (To find the phlebostatic axis point, measure the height of the chest wall and divide by two. This point is also described as being located at the midaxillary line and level with the right atrium.)

5. When patient lies in a left or right lateral position, level transducer zero port with midsternum or spinal column.

6. Use an arterial line, whenever possible, to draw blood samples. Continuous blood sampling through the PA or RA ports causes fibrin to

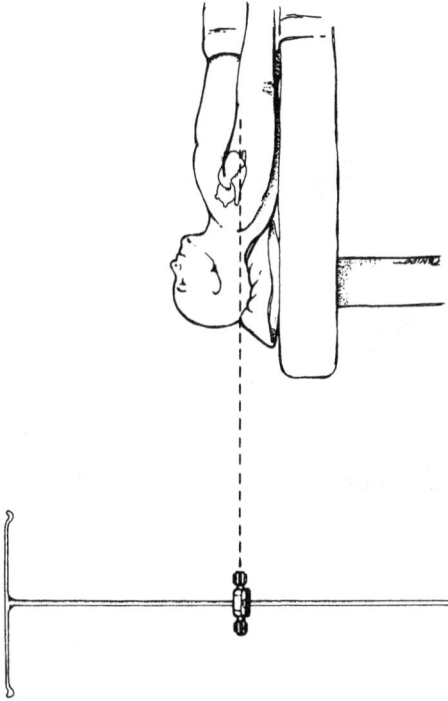

Figure 3.1 Zero Port Level with Phlebostatic Axis

accumulate and may eventually damp tracings. It is not recommended that blood cultures be drawn through PA or arterial lines due to possible false diagnosis of lacteremia.

7. Use PA distal port for drawing mixed venous blood *ONLY*, or if there is no arterial line available for taking blood samples. Do not draw blood for tests from the PA port whose results may be altered by heparin (e.g., PT, PTT).

8. Wear gloves when withdrawing blood specimens to protect both patient and nurse.

9. Flush catheter and stopcocks after taking blood samples.

10. Do not inject medicines through catheter unless absolutely necessary. Use venous infusion or proximal ports only.

11. Change dressing daily;

12. Notify the physician in the event of any of the following:
    a. Change in waveforms
    b. Waveform becomes unobtainable
    c. Continuous wedging is suspected

d. Pressure parameters deviate from acceptable range

e. Catheter begins to leak (especially if it leaks into the dressing during cardiac output injections)

f. Lines damp frequently

g. Clots are aspirated when blood samples are drawn through the catheter

13. Keep the pressure tubings and stopcocks free of air and clots.

14. In the event that the balloon ruptures, close the port, tape it shut, and indicate on the tape that the balloon has broken. Notify MD.

15. Ensure that all catheter connections are tight, and that the catheter is taped securely to the skin near the insertion site.

16. If an armboard is used, remove it at least every 8 hours and permit as much range of motion as catheter placement will allow.

17. Avoid stretching the catheter body (can cause the thermistor wires to break).

18. To avoid inadvertently leaving the catheter wedged, always take readings in this sequence:

first: PAW
second: PA
third: RA

19. When a transfer pack is used, limit the fluid in it to 100 ml (to reduce risk of fluid overload). The flush volume infused should be estimated every 8–12 hours. Fast flush system, release solution at the rate of 1.5 ml per second. Limit length of time used to clear the catheter to 2–3 seconds.

20. *Maintain strict asepsis* (see table 3.1).

B. Potential Complications Postinsertion

1. Infection

Symptoms

a. *Local infection* around insertion site: redness, swelling, exudate

b. *Systemic infection*: unexplained fever; abnormal blood, urine, or sputum cultures; abnormal CBC/differential

Table 3.1 CDC Guidelines for the Prevention of Infections Related to Intravascular Pressure-monitoring Systems[a]

Component	Recommendation	Category[b]
Flush solution	Change every 24 hours	I
Chamber dome	Change every 48 hours	II
Tubing and continuous flow device	Change every 48 hours	II
Transducer disinfection between different patients	High level disinfection with chemical agent or sterilize with ethylene oxide	I
Transducer disinfection during prolonged use by a single patient	No recommendation	No recommendation

[a]From Centers for Disease Control. Guidelines for prevention of infections related to intravascular pressure-monitoring systems. Atlanta: *Infection Control* 3, 1982: 68.
[b]Category I, strongly recommended for adoption and strongly supported by well-designed and controlled clinical studies; category II, moderately recommended for adoption and supported by highly suggestive clinical studies.

Cause

The longer the catheter is indwelling, the greater the risk of infection. To minimize this risk, whenever possible leave the catheter in no longer than 72 hours.

Action

If infection is suspected when the catheter is removed, culture the catheter tip and any exudate from around the insertion site.

2. Displacement of Catheter

Forward displacement: the catheter may wedge spontaneously: therefore, monitor pressures and waveforms constantly. When a continuous wedge is suspected, there is imminent danger of infarcting a portion of the vascular tree; the catheter must be repositioned. Be sure you are monitoring PA (RA sometimes looks similar to wedge).

Actions

a. Have the patient turn, cough, or (if an antecubital insertion) extend the arm out perpendicular to the body.

b. If this is not successful, pull the catheter back 3 to 4 cm.[a] *DO NOT* inflate the balloon or hand flush the PA lumen.

Backward displacement: after the balloon is deflated, the catheter tip may recoil. At times, it may recoil back into the right ventricle and precipitate dysrhythmias. Waveforms will show RV. Slight recoil will result in failure to wedge. In this instance, waveforms will be PA with balloon inflated.

Actions

a. Inflate the balloon and advance the catheter an additional 2 to 3 cm.[a]

b. If dysrhythmias persist, RN should withdraw catheter to RA.

3. Hemorrhage

Symptoms

a. Hemoptysis

---

[a]MD does this; RN can do if covered by written hospital protocol.

b. Signs of shock, a sudden drop in HCT and Hgb
c. Local swelling and discoloration
d. Patient may experience chest pain; is at risk for myocardial infarct because of decreased Hgb (O_2 to heart muscle)

Causes

a. Pulmonary artery perforation
b. Perforation of myocardium
c. Bleeding into groin

Actions

a. Apply compression with manual pressure or sandbags.
b. Transfusion and/or immediate surgery may be required.

4. Pulmonary Thromboembolism

Symptoms range from none to

a. Unexplained dyspnea, restlessness, chest pain
b. Tachycardia, hypotension

c. Shock, cyanosis

Cause

Clots form or migrate to the main pulmonary artery or one of its branches.

Actions

a. Confirm by ventilation-perfusion lung scan.
b. Treat with anticoagulants and correct the predisposing cause.

5. Air Embolism (from ruptured balloon)

6. Pneumothorax

SECTION 4

Measurement of Cardiac Output

A. Cardiac Output (CO)

1. Definition: The volume of blood ejected by the left ventricle in 1 minute.

Normal resting CO = 4–8 liters/min

$$CO = HR \times SV$$

CO = cardiac output
HR = heart rate
SV = stroke volume

2. Uses

a. To assess overall cardiac status, especially left ventricular performance

b. To evaluate cardiac response to therapy

3. Three Factors Affecting Stroke Volume

a. *Preload:* The length to which myocardial fibers are stretched at the end of diastole. As preload (fiber length) increases, the tension of the myocardial muscle increases, leading to increased force of contraction, which leads to increased stroke volume. However, there is a level after which any further stretching of the fibers leads to decreased or no improvement in stroke volume. Left and right ventricular preload can be measured clinically: left ventricular preload measured by PAW.

PAW $\pm$[a] left atrial pressure = LVDP

CVP $\pm$ right atrial pressure = RVDP

b. *Afterload:* The amount of resistance against which the ventricle ejects its content. As afterload increases, less volume is ejected, which leads to decreased stroke volume. Left and right ventricular

---

[a] $\pm$ = approximately equal to.

afterload can be approximated clinically by systemic and pulmonary vascular resistances, respectively (see appendix for formulas).

c. *Contractility:* The inherent ability of the myocardial cell to contract. It is not directly measurable clinically.

4. Cardiac Index (CI)

Definition: The volume of cardiac output per square meter of body surface area per minute. Cardiac index standardizes cardiac output between individuals by eliminating differences in height and weight. Treatment is usually based on cardiac index.

Normal CI (healthy, younger, resting patient) = 3.2–5.2 liters/min/m^2

$$CI = CO \div BSA$$

    CI = *cardiac index*
    CO = *cardiac output*
    BSA = *body surface area*

B. Causes of *Low* Cardiac Output

1. Valve disorders (as in stenosis or insufficiency)
2. Increased peripheral vascular resistance
3. Decreased cardiac function (as in ischemic heart disease, acute myocardial infarction, cardiomyopathies, cardiogenic shock), post-coronary artery bypass graft
4. Poor filling of the left ventricle (hypovolemia, abnormally fast or slow heart rate)

C. Causes of *High* Cardiac Output

1. Increased physical activity
2. AV shunting
3. Increased metabolic state (as in hyperthyroid, fever, tachycardia)
4. Pulmonary edema
5. Anemia
6. Mild hypertension with a wide pulse pressure

D. Treatment to Increase Cardiac Output

1. Increase stroke volume by increasing contractility; e.g., give cardiotonic drugs.
2. Increase diastolic volume; e.g., give fluids.
3. Change the heart rate; e.g., decrease or increase via pacemaker, medication.
4. Decrease peripheral resistance; e.g., afterload reduction: give diuretics and/or vasodilators.

E. Computing Cardiac Output by Thermodilution

1. Principle

Computing cardiac output by thermodilution is based on the principle that if

   a. You have an unknown amount of liquid at a known temperature (blood flow), and

b. You inject into this a known amount of another liquid that is at a known (but different) temperature (injectate), and

c. You assume that complete mixing of the two liquids will result in a specific period of time, then

d. The amount of the unknown liquid can be deduced from the amount of change in temperature (dilution curve). From this, the cardiac output is derived.

2. Points to Remember

a. Because the injectate must be injected into the RA, the RA lumen must open into the RA. Since the thermodilution probe is located near the PA lumen, it is vital that the PA lumen be in the PA. The solution must pass through both the tricuspid and pulmonic valves to mix adequately. *Displacement of the catheter will cause inaccuracy.*

b. If chilled, prefilled syringes are used, they must sit in an iced water solution for at least 20 minutes immediately prior to use. When the

5% D/W is injected, the temperature must not exceed 4°C. (Temperature of syringes can be measured by a probe from the output computer.)

c. When handling the syringes filled with injectate, DO NOT TOUCH the barrel of the syringe (will cause an erroneous reading from body heat that is conducted into the 5% D/W).

d. When injecting the 5% D/W, do it smoothly and rapidly (within 4 seconds). Slower injection time may cause the computer to reject the reading or may provide inaccurate readings.

e. Double check the volume of each syringe to ensure that the same amount of solution is injected each time. A smaller volume will result in a higher CO reading.

f. All PA catheters do not contain the same amount of liquid volume; therefore, it is important to note, per manufacturer's instructions, the value of the constant to correct the computer.

g. Consider the type of IV fluids (e.g., dopamine or hyperal versus 5% D/W) that are indwelling in the proximal line through which you inject for measurement of CO. It may be necessary to clear the line of IV solutions that could be harmful when followed by rapid CO injectates.

h. Ensure that all electrical components are connected and calibrated. Since these components differ in use between makes and models, refer to the manufacturer's literature.

3. Supplies

a. Thermodilution computer with power source

b. Cable to connect the PA catheter to the thermodilution computer

c. Five to 10, 10 ml syringes[b] prefilled with the *exact* amount of sterile 5% D/W that is required

d. One syringe with barrel removed, to hold computer thermistor probe

e. Small sterile basin filled with sterile 5% D/W, to hold syringes

---

[b]Five ml and 3 ml syringes may be used with proper computation on constants set on the computer.

f. Large basin filled with crushed ice, to hold small basin and syringes

g. Strip recorder with connecting cable, to record dilution curve (optional)

4. Procedure

a. Carry out procedure under strict sterile technique.

b. Determine that the catheter tip is located in one of the main branches of the pulmonary artery and not wedged (check pressure and waveform). The balloon must be *deflated*.

c. With the thermodilution computer set for performing the test,[c] connect the first syringe of 5% D/W injectate to the RA port (proximal lumen) and inject the solution smoothly in the allotted 4 seconds. The entire amount must be injected.

d. Wait for the computer to display the cardiac output; record the result.

e. At 1 minute intervals repeat steps c. and d. above. Measure three cardiac outputs, discard #1, and average #2 and #3. (The first result often is erroneous because the catheter is filled with fluid at body temperature.)

f. Average outputs within a 10% range of each other. (Some abnormal states, e.g., atrial fibrillation, frequent ventricular ectopics, produce cardiac outputs not within a 10% range.)

Table 4.1 Implications of Cardiac Index Readings

CI	Implications
2.0–2.2	Onset of forward failure
1.5–2.0	Cardiogenic shock
Under 1.5	Grave prognosis

5. Closed system cardiac output measurement (as per manufacturer's instructions)

F. Causes of Error in Cardiac Output Measurement

1. Faulty technique (e.g., too little injectate in the syringes or injectate loss during injection) will result in a *false high error.*

2. If the injectate is too warm (because of slow injection or handling the syringe barrel), the result will be a *false low reading.*

3. Incorrect constants set on computer will result in *false (low or high)* readings.

SECTION 5

Waveforms and Pressures

A. Scales and Speeds

1. Pressure Values

Pressure values can be obtained by measuring the actual pressure waveforms (pressure complexes) that are recorded on graph paper or from digital readouts. The preferred method is to use the values obtained from the tracings because:

a. This allows you to survey the actual pressure complexes. The digital readout selects a time interval and averages waveforms, which may introduce false low information (because inspiration or movement can occur).

b. Measuring the actual pressure waveforms provides the most reliable and comprehensive data.

c. Pressure tracings are routinely filed in the chart, become part of the permanent record, and thus can be referred to at a later time.

Note: Because pressure tracings become part of the patient's permanent record, each strip must be documented with the patient's name, the date, time, scale, and paper speed if other than the standard 25 mm/second speed is used.

2. Graph Paper

Graph paper is divided vertically into 10 major grids or boxes per channel (figure 5.1). Each major box is subdivided into five minor boxes. Pressures are determined by waveform placement on the vertical axis. Time/duration is derived from the horizontal axis.

Graph paper is commonly seen for both 2-channel and 4-channel monitoring equipment. The 2-channel paper has two grid columns, and the 4-channel paper has four grid columns.

3. Pressure Scales

Because right and left heart pressures range from low to high, different pressure scales are used to help obtain the most accurate evaluations of recorded pressures. For low pressures, select a low scale. If pressures are high, use a higher scale.

When pressures are higher than the scale, the pressure complexes will "top out" (figure 5.2).

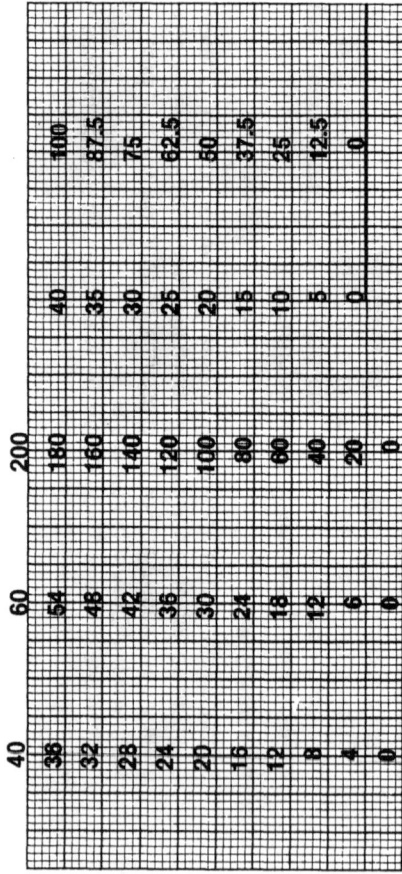

scale 40/10	60/10	200/10	40/8	100/8
40	60	200	40	100
36	54	180	40	100
32	48	160	35	87.5
28	42	140	30	75
24	36	120	25	62.5
20	30	100	20	50
16	24	80	15	37.5
12	18	60	10	25
8	12	40	5	12.5
4	6	20	0	0
0	0	0		

Figure 5.1   Graph Paper with Scales.

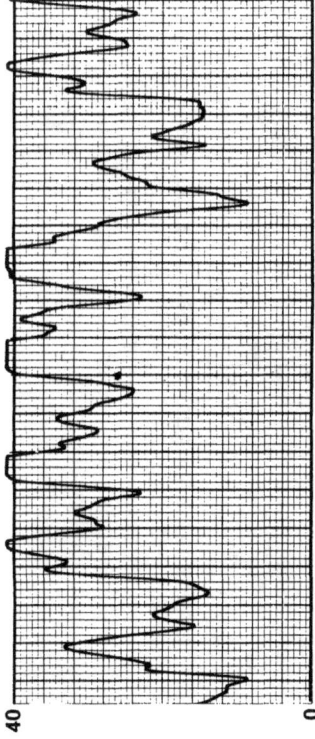

Figure 5.2   PA Pressure Topping Out at Scale 40/10.
Pulmonary artery systolic (PAS) cannot be determined from this
strip. Pulmonary artery diastolic (PAD) = 26 mm Hg.

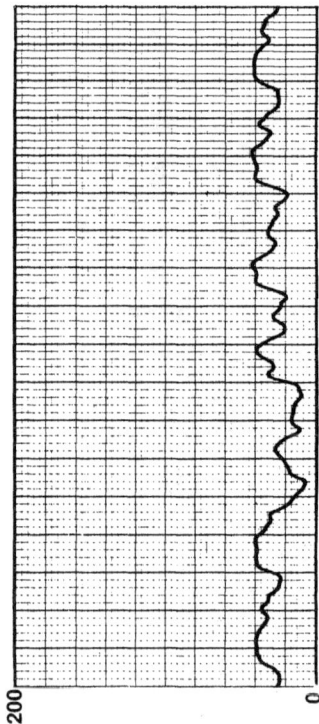

Figure 5.3   PA Pressure if Figure 5.2 Read on a 200 Scale.

PAS = 42 mm Hg. PAD is difficult to obtain accurately from this strip. Diastolic pressure *appears* lower than in figure 5.2, because the 200 scale does not measure this pressure as accurately as does the 60 scale.

When pressures are much lower than the scale being used, inaccurate pressure readings can result because the PA pressure complex is mistaken for wedge or RA waveforms.

Figure 5.3 shows PA pressure if figure 5.2 is read on a 200 scale.

4. Monitor Scales

a. *Hewlett-Packard 4-Channel Monitor Scales*

Scales on this machine are 30, 60, and 200. The 60 scale can be calibrated for either 40/0 or 60/0. For most PA pressures, any of these scales can be used. The 200 scale is usually calibrated for 200/0 and is used commonly for monitoring arterial pressures, although high pressure states, like pulmonic hypertension, may necessitate using the 200/0 scale for PA pressures.

Because this monitoring unit uses all 10 vertical grids to indicate 0-40, 0-60, or 0-200, pressures are derived by dividing the systolic and diastolic components by a factor of 10 (see figure 5.1).

b. *2-Channel Monitor Scales*

Some of the newer bedside monitoring units utilize only two channels, and the scales may differ. For instance, the pressure scales may be 20/0, 40/0, 100/0, and 200/0 and have a factor of 8 because only 8 of the major boxes are used in measuring pressures (see figure 5.1). Here, the 40 and 100 scales are most useful in PA pressure monitoring.

5. Paper Speed

Pressure monitoring units usually have a selection of paper speeds that range from 5 mm/second to 50 mm/second. Standard speed is 25 mm/second, the same as EKG paper. The slower the graph paper moves past the stylus, the closer the pressure complexes are to each other. At the slower speeds, the pressure complexes are also narrower than at standard speed.

Slower-than-standard speed is used often when there is slight respiratory variation. By tracing the pressure complexes in close proximity to each other, it is easier to identify the true end-expiratory waveforms for proper pressure measurement. Faster speeds are used to identify waveform components.

Faster-than-standard speed results in the opposite distortions. The pressure complexes are expanded in width, and the distance between each waveform is increased (figure 5.4).

B. Pressure Complexes

1. Measurement

Pressure complexes are correctly measured at the end of expiration, when the intrathoracic pressure is closest to a state of equilibrium with the intraventricular pressures. Inspiration causes a fall in the baseline pressure (respiratory variation). End of expiration will be found two or three complexes before inspiration (figure 5.5).

Hint: To evaluate the pressures:

a. Put a bar over the two or three pressure complexes that are most similar.

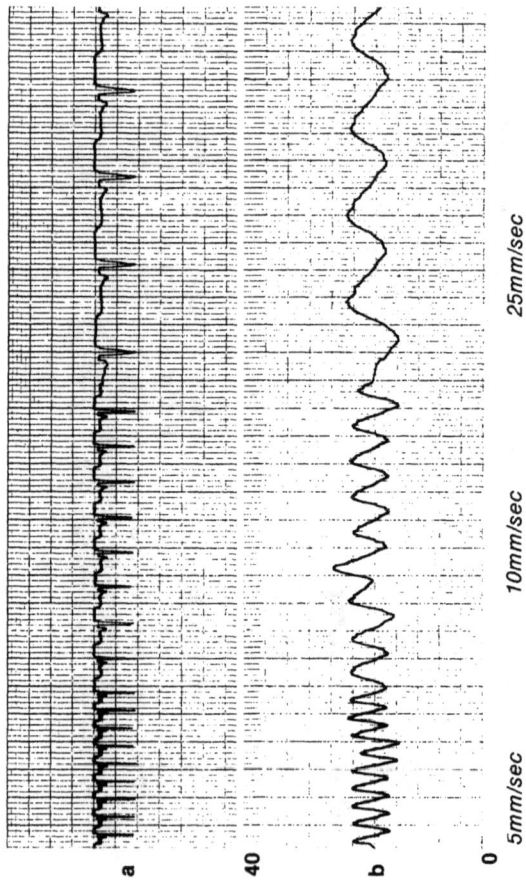

a

b

40

0

5mm/sec   10mm/sec   25mm/sec

Figure 5.4 EKG and PA Tracing at Speeds of 5, 10, and 25 mm/second, on a Scale of 40.
   a. EKG
   b. PA Tracing

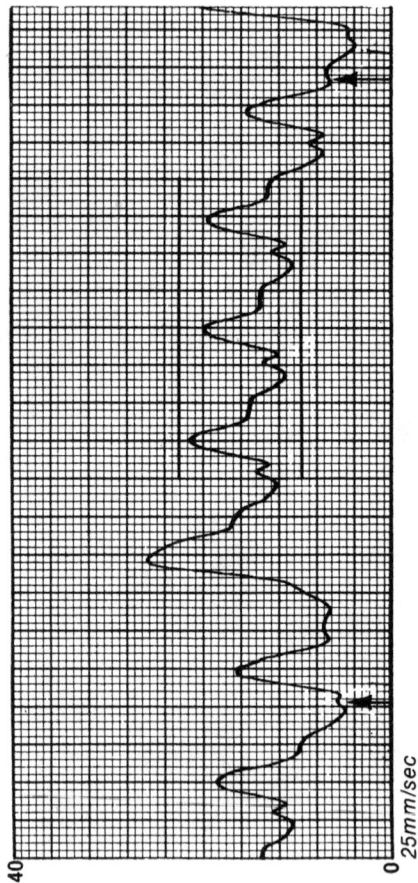

Figure 5.5   PA Tracing with Respiratory Variation.
Arrows indicate onset of inspiration. Complexes barred over are
end-expiratory. PA is 20/11 mm Hg.

0   25mm/sec

b. Note the pressures at the peak of each complex and average them. This is the *systolic* pressure.

c. Do the same for the troughs. This is the *diastolic* pressure.

d. Accurate pressure evaluation when sustained dysrhythmias are present may require averaging pressure complexes from several waveforms (see figure 5.6).

e. Mechanical ventilators that deliver positive end-expiratory pressure (PEEP) will cause PA systolic and diastolic pressure to go up during PEEP delivery. Correct by measuring 2 or 3 complexes before the rise. It is not necessary or advisable to take the patient off the ventilator (see figure 5.7).

2. Combining Scales

When a pressure is too high to be read on a 40 scale, a combination of 40 and 200 scales is used to determine diastolic and systolic waves (figures 5.8 and 5.9).

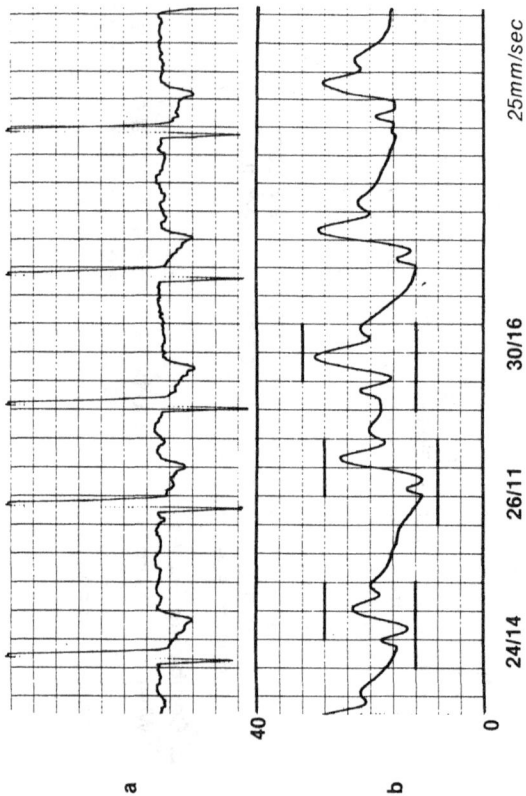

a

b

24/14   26/11   30/16   25mm/sec

40

0

Figure 5.6 Atrial Fibrillation: PA Pressures Vary with RV Stroke Volume.
 a. EKG.
 b. Waveform. Averaging pressure complexes gives a mean PAS of 27 and a mean PAD of 14 (27/14 mm Hg).

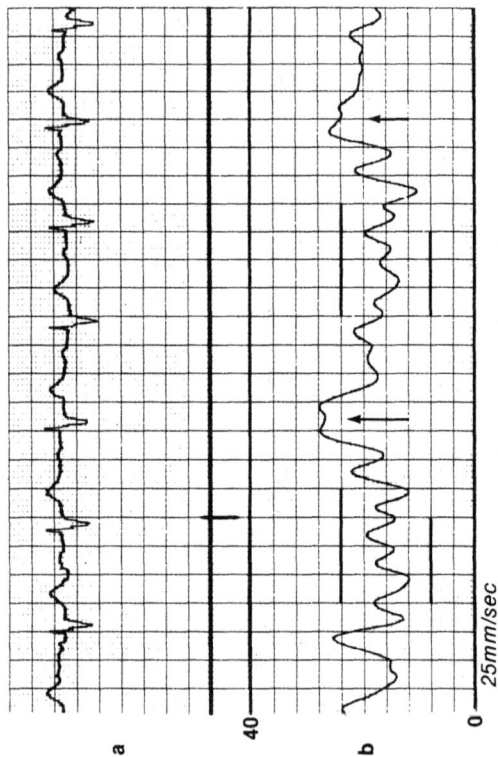

25mm/sec

Figure 5.7 PAW with PEEP on a Mechanical Ventilator.
   a. EKG.
   b. Waveform (arrows indicate PEEP. PAW = 16 mm Hg).

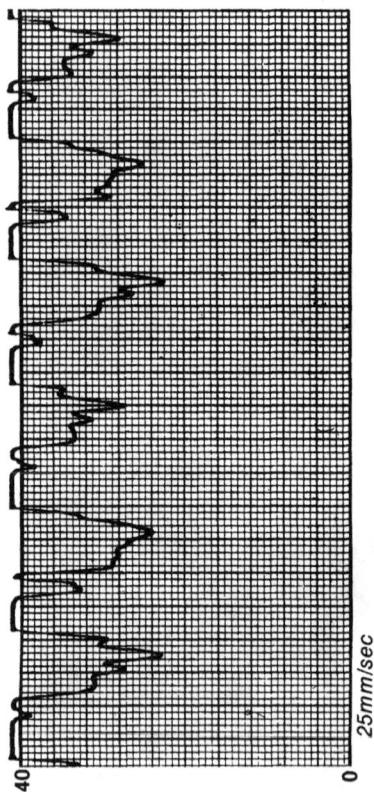

25mm/sec

Figure 5.8 Combining Scales, Scale 40/10.
Square tops indicate systolic artifactual blocking. Although the PAD can be accurately taken from this strip, the PAS cannot. A higher scale is needed. PAD = 27 mm Hg. Abnormal tracing shows increased PA pressure.

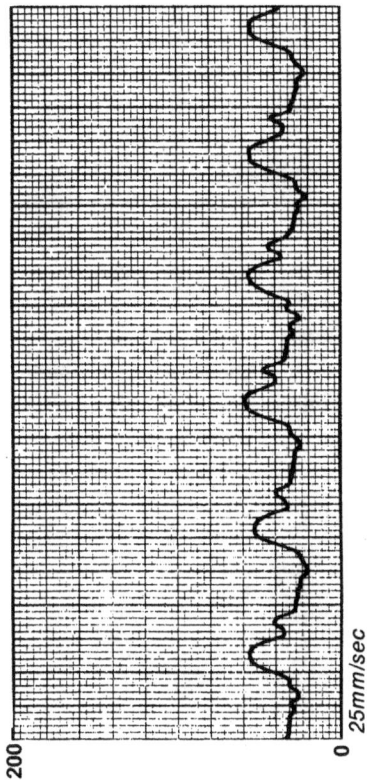

200

0 *25mm/sec*

Figure 5.9 Combining Scales, Scale 200/10.
PA pressure same as in figure 5.8. Systolic can be read accurately. PAS = 56 mm Hg. Diastolic is not read as accurately as on 40 scale: PAD = 20 mm Hg. Combined pressure of figures 5.8 and 5.9: PAS = 56, PAD = 27 (56/27 mm Hg).

3. Measuring Waveform Components (figure 5.10)

a. *Absolute*: from 0 scale to top of wave.

b. *Relative*: from baseline to waveform to top of waveform.

c. Components may be measured either way (absolute or relative), but method must be indicated.

$$A^a = A \text{ wave } \textit{absolute}$$
$$A^r = A \text{ wave } \textit{relative}$$
$$V^a = V \text{ wave } \textit{absolute}$$
$$V^r = V \text{ wave } \textit{relative}$$

d. A and V waves are normally very similar in height. When compared with each other, a difference of 10 mm or more suggests an abnormality.

e. The A wave follows atrial contraction. The V wave follows ventricular contraction.

f. Normal values (appendix 5) are guides for relative values.

4. Digital Readout Errors

With respiratory variation, the digital readout and printout will average pressures and frequently record a *false low* error. For this reason, it is important to determine what the end-expiratory pressures are. In figure 5.11, the digital printout gives a value of 30/4 mm Hg for the PA pressure, but the correct end-expiratory pressure is 28/16 mm Hg. The erroneous printout of 30/4 mm Hg indicates hypovolemia, but the actual PA pressure of 28/16 mm Hg is in the normal range. The treatment for hypovolemia is to increase volume with normal saline or volume expanders. If volume was increased in a damaged heart with a normal pressure of 28/16 mm Hg, it could precipitate cardiac failure.

C. Waveforms and Components

The pressure waveforms correspond with the EKG (figure 5.12). The EKG events are electrical and precede the mechanical events of the pressure tracings.

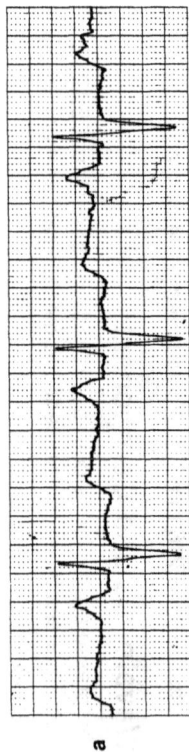

a

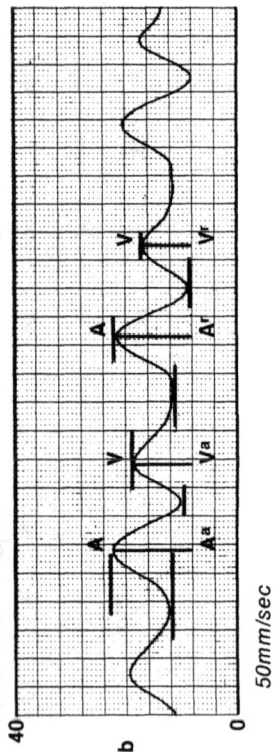

b

50mm/sec

40

0

Figure 5.10 Measuring PAW Waveform Components.

a. EKG.

b. Waveform. A^a = 22 mm Hg, V^a = 18 mm Hg, A^r = 10 mm Hg, V^r = 8 mm Hg. Mean PAW = 15 mm Hg.

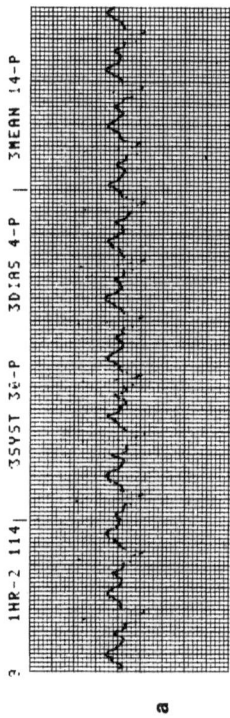

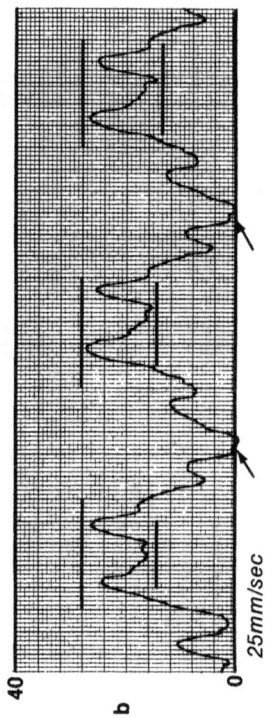

Figure 5.11 Digital Readout Error.
   a. EKG.
   b. Waveform. Arrows indicate onset of inspiration. Note digital printout at top of strip. It indicatesa PA pressure of 30/4 mm Hg. Measured end-expiratory pressure is 28/16 mm Hg.

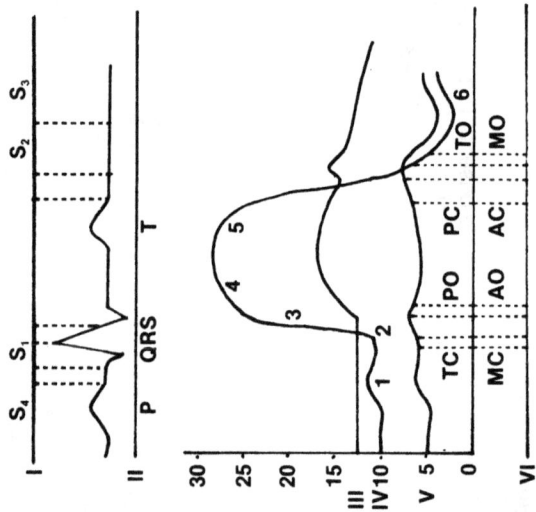

Figure 5.12   Cardiac Cycle: Heart Sounds, EKG, Waveforms, Valvular Motion.

I. Heart sounds
II. EKG
III. Pulmonary artery waveform
IV. Right ventricular waveform
  1. Atrial systole
  2. RV end-diastole
  3. Isovolumetric contraction
  4. Ventricular ejection
  5. Isovolumetric relaxation
  6. RV early diastole
V. Right atrial waveform with A, C, and V waves
VI. Valvular motion

TC = tricuspid closing
MC = mitral closing
PO = pulmonic opening
AO = aortic opening
PC = pulmonic closing
AC = aortic closing
TO = tricuspid opening
MO = mitral valve opening

1. Right Atrial Waveform

These components are seen in right atrial (RA) and pulmonary artery wedge (PAW) waveforms, which reflect left atrial (LA) activity (figure 5.13).

2. Right Ventricular Waveform

The right ventricular (RV) pressure complex is rectangular in shape and starts with or slightly after the QRS (figure 5.14).

a. *Atrial systole.* The "shoulder" represents a slight increase in pressure and is the result of the so-called "atrial kick."

b. *End diastole.* The period between atrial systole and the beginning of ventricular systole when the pressure represents right ventricular end-diastolic pressure and is a determinant of the potential stretch/stroke volume of the right ventricle.

c. *Isovolumetric contraction.* Pressure rises in the ventricle as muscle fibers increase tension and volume remains constant between closed tricuspid and pulmonic valves.

d. *Ventricular ejection.* Increased pressure in the right ventricle opens the pulmonic valve, and rapid ejection occurs.

e. *Isovolumetric relaxation.* Pulmonic valve closes, and tension decreases in ventricle as muscle fibers relax. Constant volume is maintained between closed AV and pulmonic valves.

f. *Early diastole.* RV pressure falls until RA pressure exceeds it and forces open the tricuspid valve, passively filling the ventricle.

3. Pulmonary Artery Waveform

The PA pressure complex appears triangular in shape and begins 15 to 20 milliseconds after the QRS (figure 5.15).

Approximately one-third of the waveform represents systole in the pulmonary artery. The remaining two-thirds represent diastole in the pulmonary artery. The dichrotic notch represents closure of the pulmonic valve. High frequency waves may be seen during diastole. They are artifactual in nature.

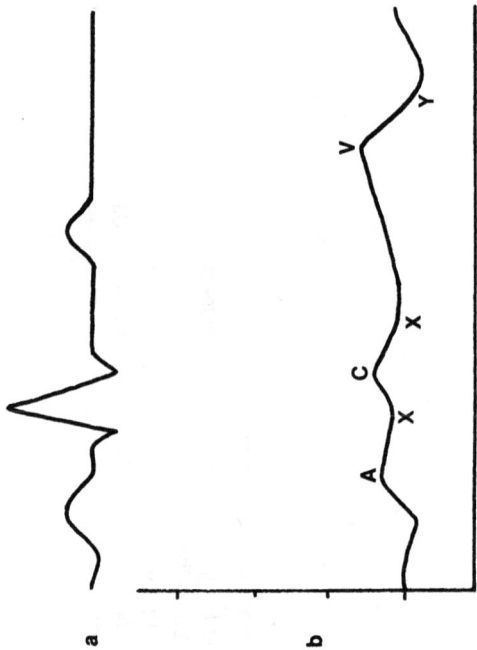

Figure 5.13 Right Atrial Waveform Components and EKG.

a. EKG

   a. A wave follows P.

   c. C wave follows R.

   v. V wave follows T.

b. RA Components

A = Mechanical atrial systole (atrial contraction).

X = Descent as pressure drops in atria (mechanical atrial diastole) and from tricuspid valve being pulled down during ventricular systole. Found on downslopes of both the A wave and the C wave.

C = Closure of valve leaflets and valvular bulging into atria. RA = tricuspid valve. LA = mitral valve (C wave is not always seen, and sometimes it notches the A wave).

V = Atrial passive filling and mechanical ventricular systole.

Y = Descent as tricuspid and mitral valves open, and atria passively empty into the ventricles.

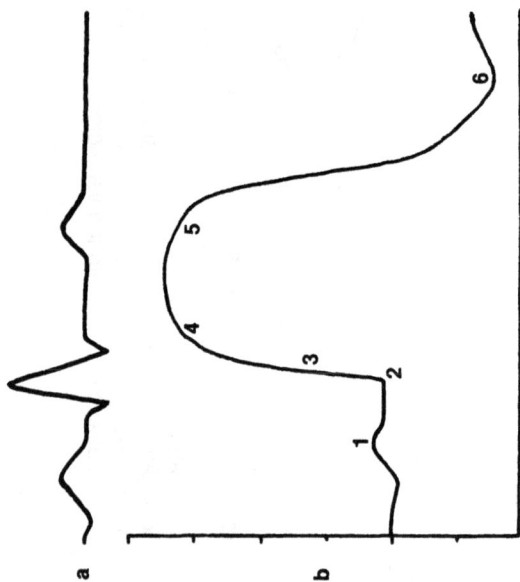

Figure 5.14 Right Ventricular Waveform Components and EKG.

a. EKG

b. RV Components: **1.** Atrial systole. **2.** End diastole. **3.** Isovolumetric contraction. **4.** Ventricular ejection. **5.** Isovolumetric relaxation. **6.** Early diastole.

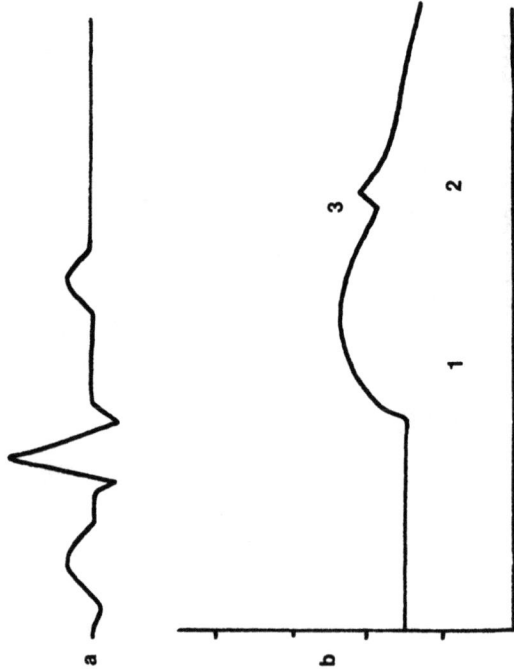

a

b

1

2

3

Figure 5.15 Pulmonary Artery Waveform Components and EKG.
a. EKG
b. PA Components: **1.** Systole. **2.** Diastole. **3.** Dichrotic notch/pulmonic valve closure.

D. Pressure Tracings

1. Right Atrial (figures 5.16-5.18)

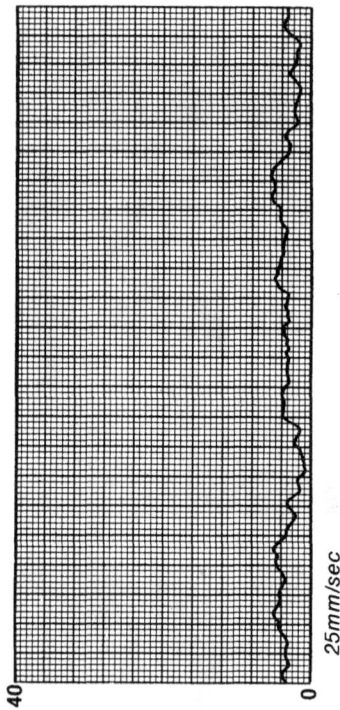

25mm/sec

Figure 5.16   Normal RA.
Mean RA pressure = 5 mm Hg (normal).

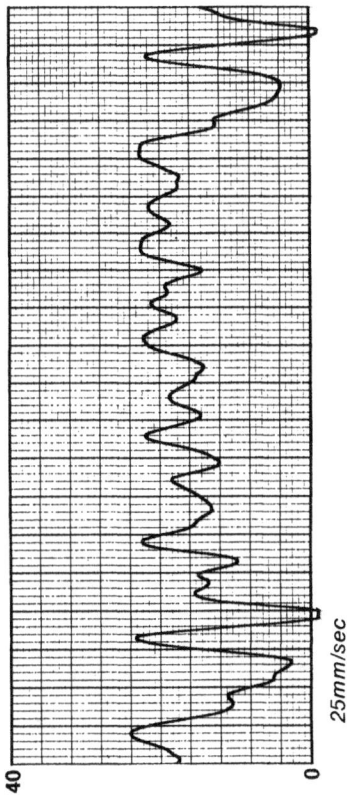

25mm/sec

Figure 5.17 Elevated RA.
Mean RA = 20 mm Hg. Right atrial failure suggests right ventricular failure, cardiac tamponade, hypervolemia, tricuspid valve stenosis, or congenital heart disease.

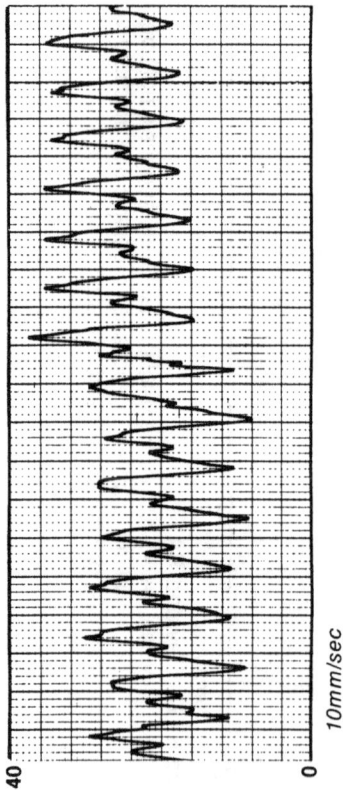

10mm/sec

Figure 5.18   Extremely Elevated RA.

Mean RA = 23 mm Hg. This tracing suggests tricuspid regurgitation (during systole, blood flows back into the right atrium through an incompetent valve). To obtain an approximation of a mean pressure, add the systolic (35) and twice the diastolic (17) pressures, and divide by 3.

$$\frac{(S + 2D)}{3} = \frac{35 + 34}{3} = 23 \text{ mm Hg}$$

2. Right Ventricular (figures 5.19-5.23)

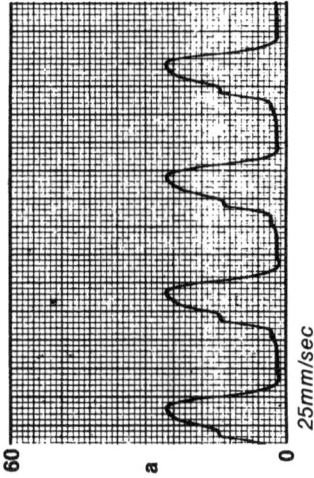

Figure 5.19 Normal RV.

RVS = 25, RVD = 3 (25/3 mm Hg). RV pressures when catheter inserted. If these pressures were present after insertion, catheter position would be incorrect.

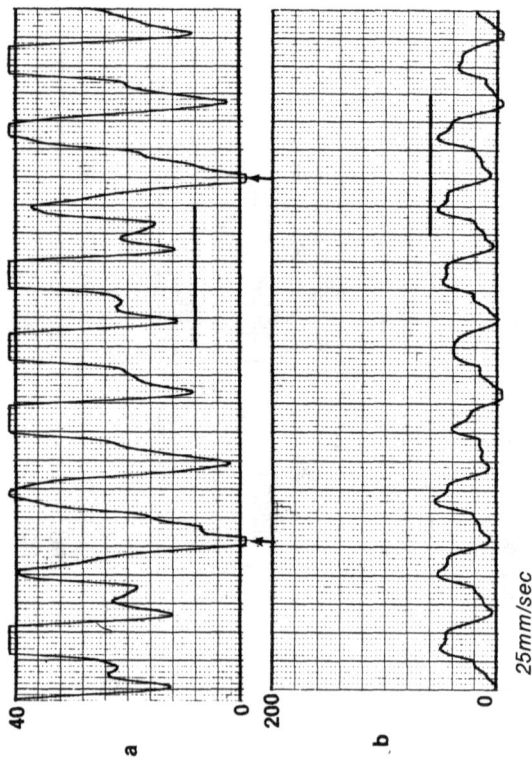

25mm/sec

Figure 5.20 Elevated RV.

a. RVD = 12 (arrows indicate inspiration).
b. RVS = 52. RV pressure of 52/12 mm Hg suggestive of right
ventricular failure.

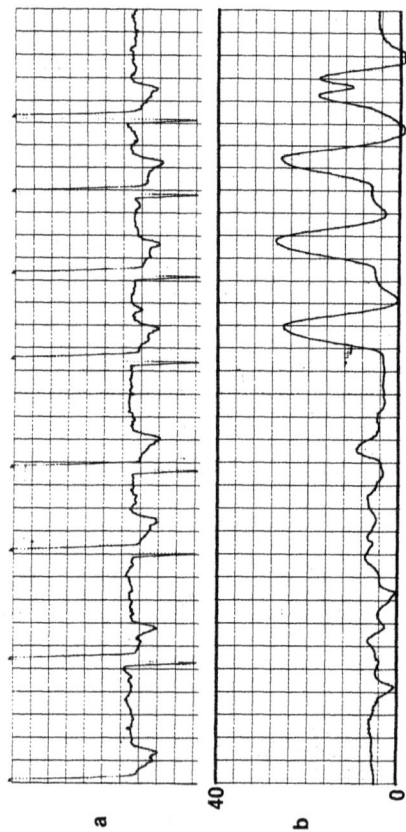

Figure 5.21 Progression of RA to RV.

a. EKG: Underlying rhythm is atrial fibrillation. Therefore, no A waves because there are no forceful atrial contractions.

b. Waveform.

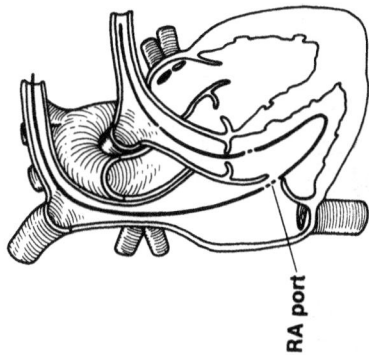

c

RA port

c. PA catheter in heart. Excess catheter is in the RA near the tricuspid valve, systole can push RA port into RV. Catheter must be pulled back into proper position. In the current position, catheter can cause dysrhythmias.

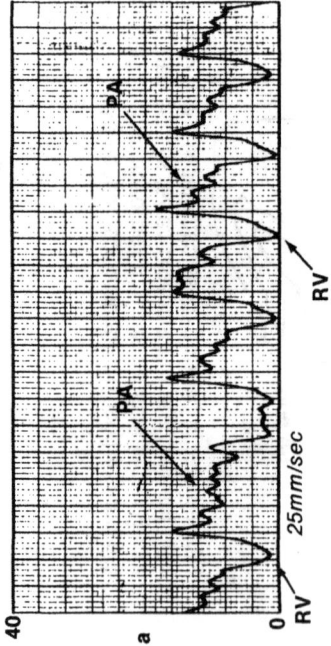

Figure 5.22 RV to PA.

a. Waveform. Catheter near pulmonic valve outflow tract of RV. PA tracing alternates between RV and PA. Systole pushes catheter into PA. In diastole, catheter falls back into RV.

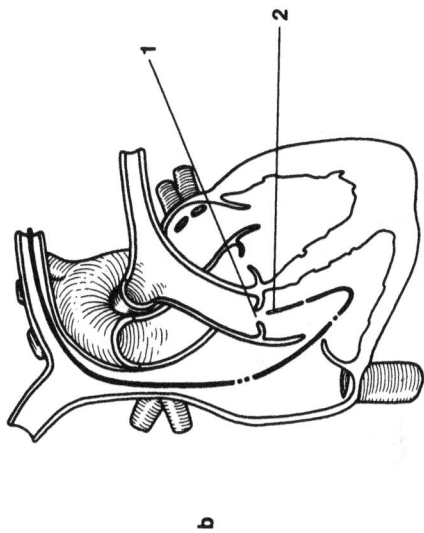

b. PA catheter tip near pulmonic valve. **1.** Pulmonic valve. **2.** PA port.

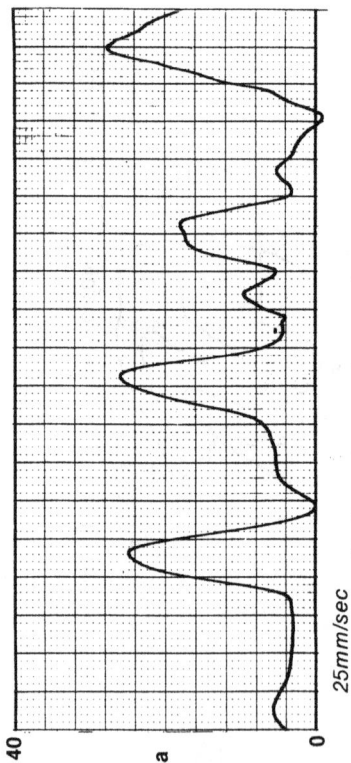

25mm/sec

Figure 5.23 RV to PA (Balloon Inflated).

a. Waveform. In the first two complexes of this tracing, the tip of the PA catheter is in RV. After the second complex the balloon is inflated, and the catheter floats forward to PA.

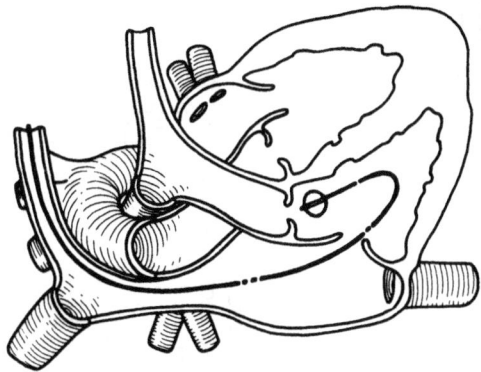

b. PA catheter tip near pulmonic valve (balloon inflated).

3. Pulmonary Artery (figures 5.24-5.26)

Figure 5.24 RV Compared to PA.

a. RV: **1.** Rectangular shape. **2.** No dichrotic notch. **3.** Steep incline with rising pressure. **4.** Steep decline in pressure. **5.** Gradual incline as blood fills right ventricle from right atrium during diastole. **6.** RVS = 25, RVD = 3 (25/3 mm Hg).

b. Normal PA: Triangular shape with dichrotic notch = pulmonic closure. Gradual decline in pressure. Decrease in pressure as pulmonary artery empties until right ventricular pressure opens pulmonic valve and creates systole. PA = 23/14 mm Hg.

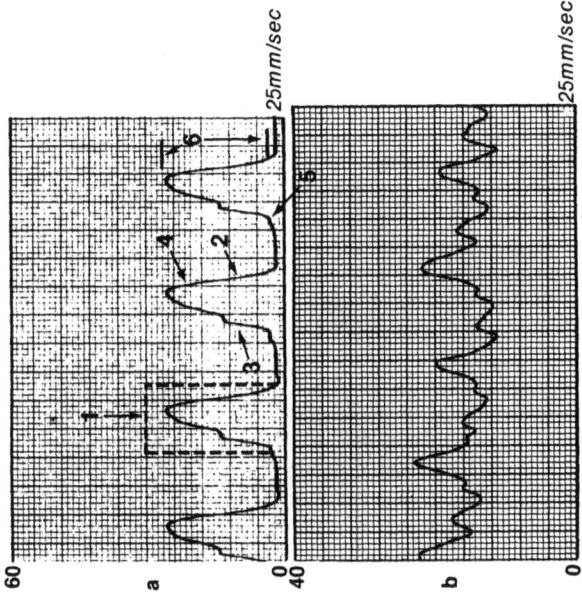

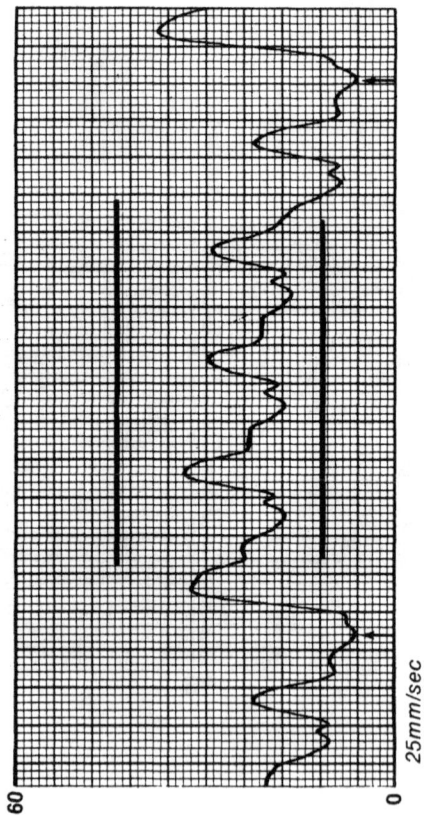

25mm/sec

Figure 5.25   Elevated PA.

PA = 30/17 mm Hg suggests mild pulmonary congestion. In a heart with preexisting right or left ventricular failure, a PAD of 16 to 20 mm Hg may be necessary to perfuse the coronary arteries. 30/17 mm Hg would be an acceptable pressure in these circumstances. Arrows indicate inspiration.

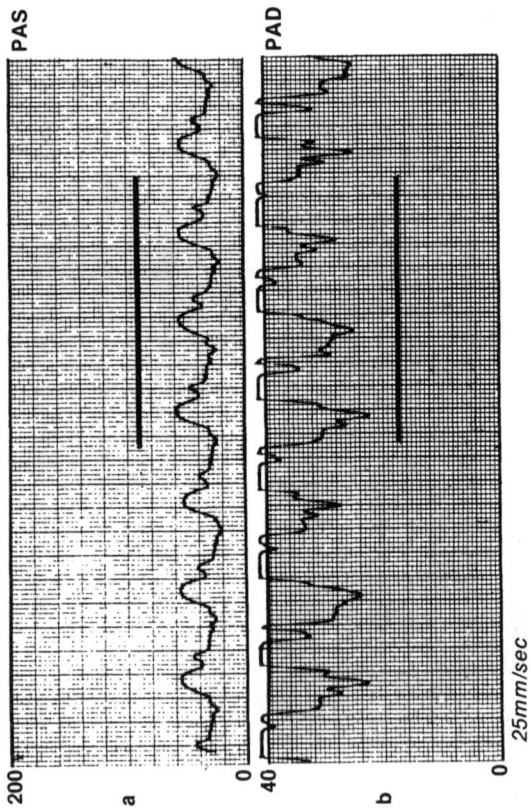

PAS

PAD

200

0
40

0

a

b

25mm/sec

Figure 5.26 Extremely Elevated PA.
Combined values PAS/PAD. PA = 56/27 mm Hg. High pressure suggests left ventricular failure or pulmonary hypertension.

4. Pulmonary Artery Wedge (figures 5.27-5.32)

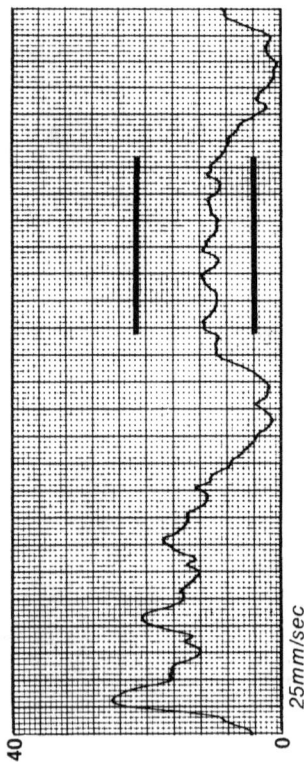

25mm/sec

Figure 5.27   Normal PAW.
Mean PAW = 10 mm Hg. Dip in the baseline is normal inspiratory variation. When recording PAW, it is advisable to demonstrate the changing PA to PAW waveforms and note amount of air required to inflate the balloon for waveform wedge.

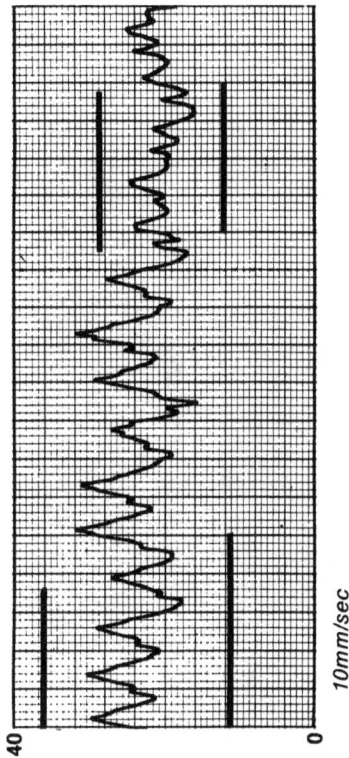

10mm/sec

Figure 5.28 PA to PAW: Elevated Pressures.
This strip shows PA waveform turning to PAW as the balloon is inflated and the PA catheter wedges. PA = 30/20 mm Hg. PAW = 20 mm Hg. These abnormally high pressures suggest left heart failure.

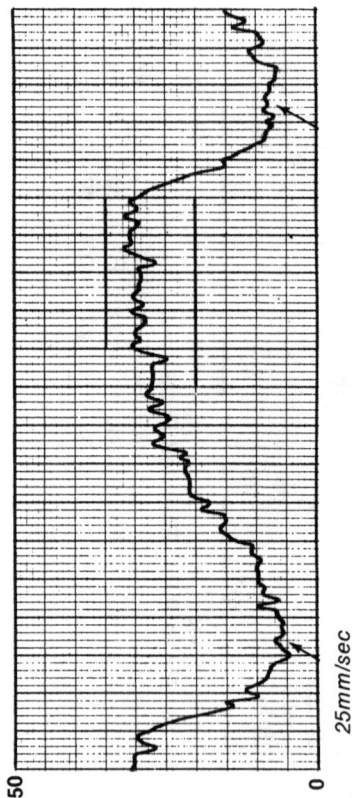

25mm/sec

Figure 5.29 Extremely Elevated PAW.

Arrows indicate respiratory variation which must be eliminated to obtain a correct reading. Mean PAW (measured correctly) = 30 mm Hg (barred segment). If low inspiratory pressure and high inspiratory pressures are averaged, the mean = 17 mm Hg (a gross error). Correct mean of 30 mm Hg favors development of pulmonary edema and requires prompt treatment.

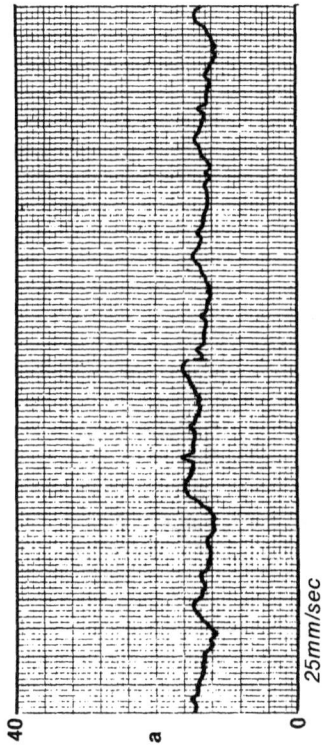

25mm/sec

Figure 5.30 Continuous Wedge

a. PA is being monitored in this strip.

b. PA catheter is in a small branch of the pulmonary artery, balloon deflated. The catheter must be withdrawn to the pulmonary artery. Damage to pulmonary tissue will result if the catheter remains continuously wedged, or if fluid is injected through the catheter.

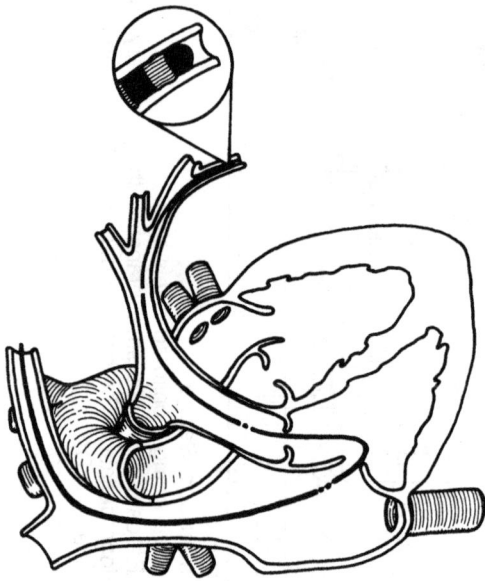

b

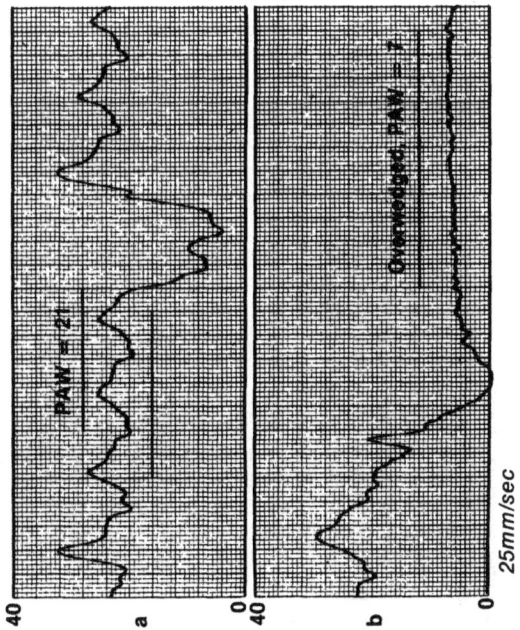

PAW = 21

Overwedged; PAW = ?

40

a

0

40

b

0

25mm/sec

SECTION 5: Waveforms and Pressures   129

Figure 5.31 Overwedged Tracing.

a. This continuous strip illustrates another common error in the use of the PA catheter. Overinflating the balloon causes "overwedging," which gives false values. A, C, and V waves are seen in PAW = 21 mm Hg.

b. Overwedged PAW of 7 mm Hg loses characteristic waveform components. Overwedging occurred when balloon was inflated beyond the 3/4 ml that was initially required to obtain PAW waveform. To wedge the catheter correctly, inflate the balloon *only* until a PAW waveform appears on the monitor.

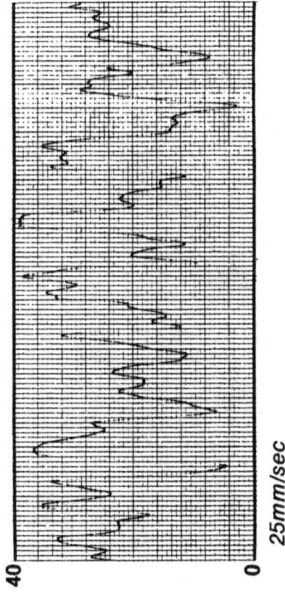

25mm/sec

Figure 5.32 Catheter Whip/Fling.
Catheter whip/fling is demonstrated in tracing by jagged, saw-tooth artifact in waveform. This suggests that the catheter position in the pulmonary artery reflects turbulence. Pressure cannot be read accurately. Whip/fling may also be due to excess tubing or patient movement.

E. Diagnostic Pressures

Data obtained from the PA catheter are of great diagnostic use, but are most reliable when corroborated with other clinical findings. Once a diagnosis is made, effectiveness of treatment often is assessed best by monitoring these same PA pressures. This section deals with abnormal states and presupposes corroborating clinical findings. Consult the bibliography for a more thorough discussion of clinical evaluation.

1. Congestive Heart Failure

a. Pulmonary venous congestion results from left ventricular dysfunction.

b. Left ventricular filling pressure is elevated and is represented by an increased PAW, which reflects an elevated LVDP.

c. An elevated A wave can sometimes be seen in the PAW. This is specific for increased left ventricular filling pressure.

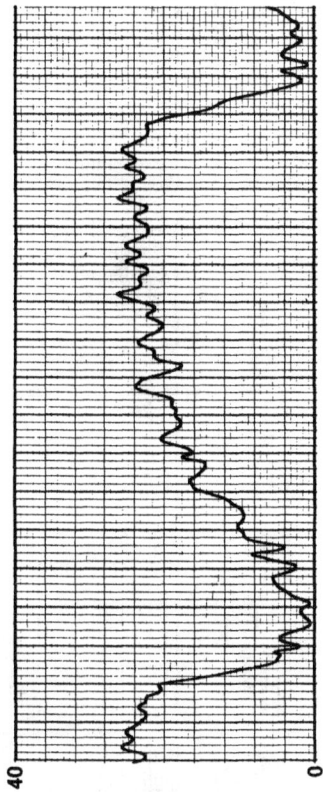

25mm/sec

Figure 5.33   PAW Tracing.
PAW = 24 mm Hg.

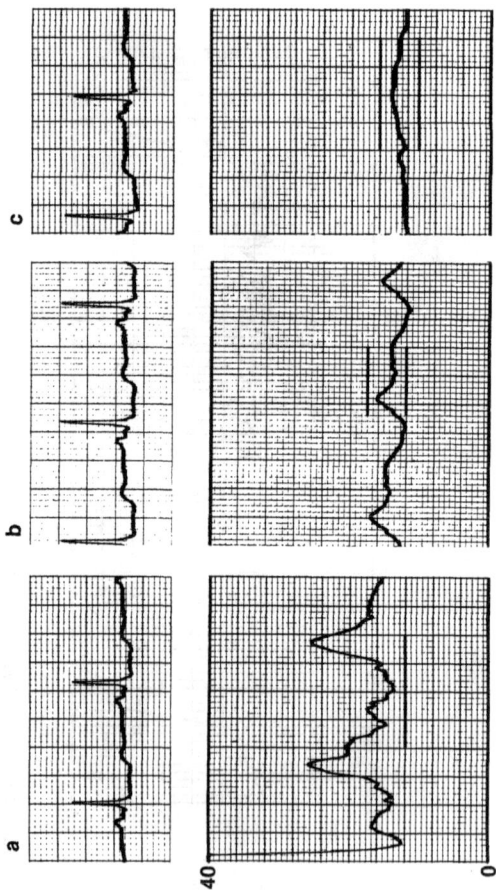

Figure 5.34 Equalized Pressures.
  a. PAD = 13 mm Hg.
  b. PAW = 13 mm Hg.
  c. RA = 13 mm Hg.

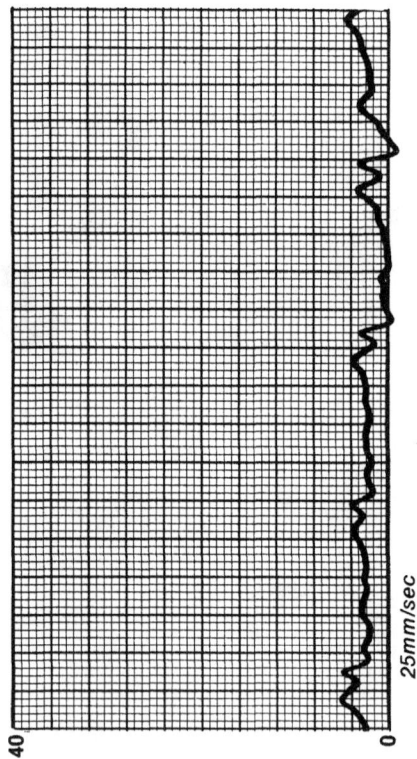

40

0

25mm/sec

Figure 5.35   PAW Tracing.
PAW = 3 mm Hg.

2. Cardiac Tamponade

a. Fluid (either serous or blood) accumulates in the pericardial sac. The ventricles can neither fill nor pump adequately.

b. Cardiac output and systemic blood pressure drop.

c. PAD, PAW, and RA equalize (RA = PAD = PAW). This condition often is fatal.

3. Hypovolemia

a. Insufficient circulating volume to maintain adequate pressures.

b. All pressures (RA, PA, PAW, systemic BP) and cardiac output are lower than normal.

c. In the uncompromised heart, the PAW may be from 4 to 6 mm Hg. In the diseased heart, the PAW may be somewhat higher. However, if the other values are depressed, suspect hypovolemia.

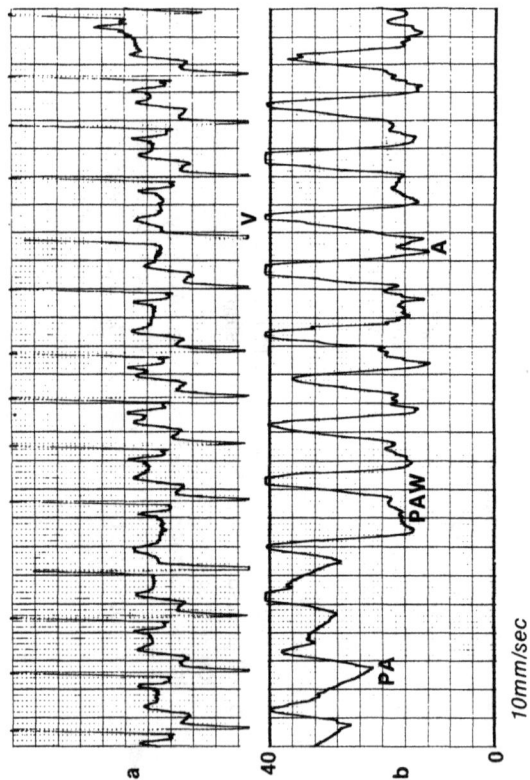

10mm/sec

Figure 5.36 PAW with V Waves.

a. EKG

b. Waveform: A^a = 19 mm Hg; V^a = 40 mm Hg; A^r = 6 mm Hg; V^r = 26 mm Hg. V waves, as compared with A waves, are grossly elevated (20 mm Hg difference in relative A and V waves). PAD is the best estimate of LVDP when mitral regurgitation is present.

4. Mitral Valve Regurgitation

a. An incompetent mitral valve will result in retrograde blood flow during ventricular systole.

b. In the chronic state, both left atrial hypertrophy and left ventricular
hypertrophy occur to compensate for the resulting loss in cardiac
output. Pulmonic pressures elevate, and eventually the right heart
fails.

c. The acute form of mitral regurgitation, as when a papillary muscle
ruptures, may quickly result in fulminating pulmonary edema and
cardiogenic shock.

d. PAW and PA pressures are elevated. The PAW may have a V wave
that lasts through mechanical ventricular systole.

e. V waves are compared to A waves. V waves that are 10 mm
greater than A waves are considered significant.

f. V wave height is determined by the amount of blood present in the
atrium at the end of diastole, the compliance of the atrium, and the
amount of blood that enters the atrium during systole.

g. Hypovolemia may prevent significant V waves even when mitral regurgitation is severe. Congestive heart failure, VSD, and mitral obstruction may cause significant V waves in the absence of mitral regurgitation.

h. When mitral regurgitation occurs, the PAD is a better measurement of LVDP than the PAW.

5. Mitral Valve Stenosis

a. Blood flow from the left atrium (LA) to the left ventricle (LV) is impeded at the mitral valve. To move the blood past the stenosed valve, the left atrium enlarges and pumps at higher than normal pressure. In this condition, PAW is greater than LVDP, and treatments must not further reduce left ventricular filling.

b. The increased LA pressure backs up through the pulmonic system and into the right heart.

c. Pulmonary vascular resistance (PVR) increases and can gradually progress to systemic levels.

d. Look for a high PAW, low cardiac output, very high pulmonic pressures, right ventricular failure, and tricuspid regurgitation.

e. Elevated and exaggerated A waves in the PAW tracing are due to the increased resistance of LV filling. Also, the Y descent of the PAW is prolonged as the result of increased resistance of passive LV filling.

6. Pulmonary Edema

a. Left ventricular failure and mitral stenosis are the most common causes of pulmonary edema, since both conditions impede the flow of blood from the lungs via the pulmonic veins. With the right heart pumping blood normally into the pulmonic vascular bed, fluid accumulates and pressure rises in the pulmonary capillaries until pulmonary edema results. If unrecognized and untreated, this condition is often fatal.

b. PAW is 30 mm Hg or higher and frequently has marked respiratory variation.

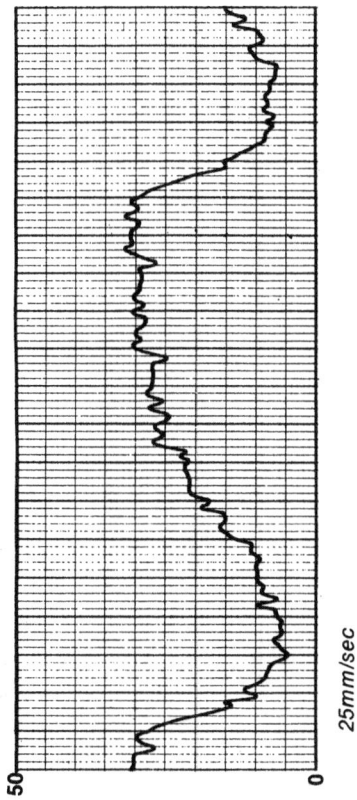

25mm/sec

Figure 5.37 PAW Tracing.

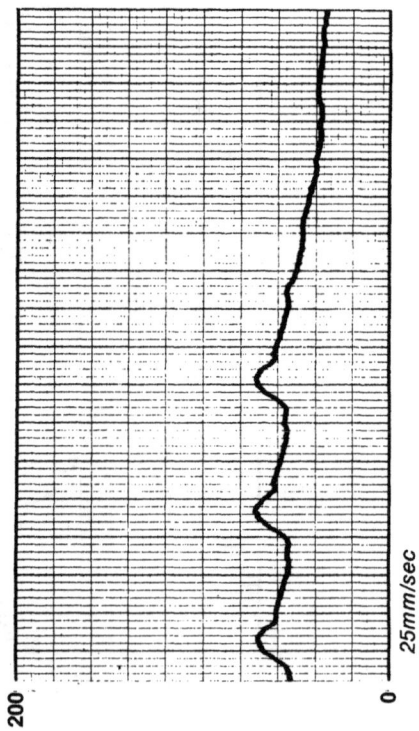

25mm/sec

Figure 5.38 PA to PAW.
PA = 67/52; mean PAW = 40 mm Hg. Elevated PAS/PAD and PAW. If difference between PAD and PAW is greater than 10 mm Hg in the absence of obstructive pulmonary disease, it is suggestive of pulmonary embolus.

Table 5.1   Implications of PAW Pressure

PAW	Implications
18-20 mg Hg	Onset of pulmonary congestion
20-25 mg Hg	Moderate pulmonary congestion
25-30 mg Hg	Severe pulmonary congestion
30 + mg Hg	Acute pulmonary congestion

With permission from Forrester, J., Chatterjee, K., and Swan, H. "Hemodynamic Monitoring in Patients with Acute Myocardial Infarction." *JAMA*, October 1, 1973:60-61.

7. Pulmonary Embolus

a. In this condition, clots form or migrate to the main pulmonary artery or one of its branches. Symptoms range from none to otherwise unexplained dyspnea, restlessness, tachycardia, hypotension, shock, cyanosis, and sudden death.

b. In the absence of pulmonary disease, when the above symptoms are seen together with a PAD of 10 mm Hg or more higher than the PAW, suspect pulmonary embolus.

8. Pulmonary Hypertension

  a. Elevated PA pressures due to pulmonary hypertension, mitral valve
     disease, left ventricular failure, left-to-right shunting (atrial or ventric-
     ular), and hypoxia (which increases PVR).

  b. PAS and PAD are elevated.

  c. PAW normal (if no left heart involvement).

9. Right Ventricular Infarct

  a. Right ventricular infarction initially results in systemic venous con-
     gestion, as opposed to initial pulmonic venous congestion of LV
     infarction.

  b. RA pressure will be elevated, equal to, or greater than the PAW.

  c. PA, CO, and systemic BP will be normal or below.

10. Septic Shock

a. Early onset is hemodynamically characterized by low pressures, low systemic vascular resistance (SVR) (resulting from peripheral vasodilation), and a high cardiac output.

b. RA, PA, and PAW will be low.

c. CO will be high because of the low SVR. This manifestation differentiates septic shock from hypovolemia.

d. As shock progresses, pressures may elevate.

11. Tricuspid Valve Regurgitation

a. Usually the result of advanced right- or left-sided heart failure or severe pulmonary hypertension, which causes the right ventricle to deteriorate and fail. The failing RV enlarges and produces regurgitation through the tricuspid valve.

b. The large retrograde blood flow (from RV back into RA) distorts the C and V waves.

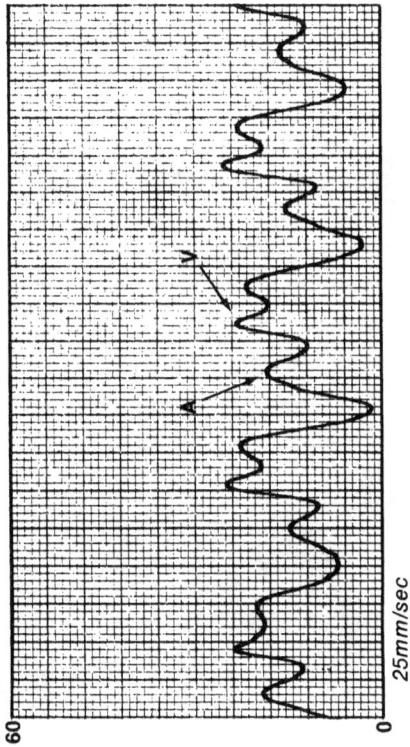

25mm/sec

Figure 5.39 **RA Tracing.**
Mean RA = 15 mm Hg. **A** = A wave. **V** = V wave.

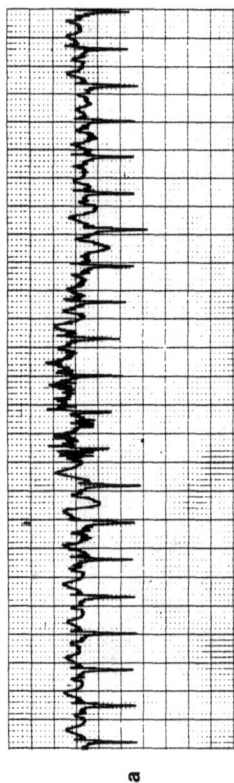
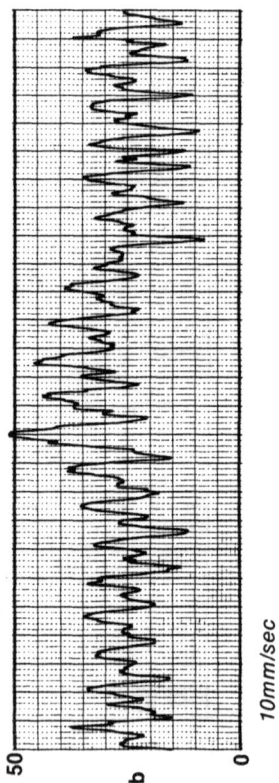

a

b

50

0

10mm/sec

Figure 5.40 RA Tracing Suggesting Tricuspid Regurgitation.
   a. EKG
   b. Waveform: Mean RA = 23 mm Hg.

12. Tricuspid Valve Stenosis

a. In this condition, blood flow from the right atrium to the right ventricle is restricted at the tricuspid valve.

b. To move blood past the stenosed valve, the right atrium must exert greater pressure, which produces giant A waves.

Appendix 1   Maintenance of Line Integrity

A. Ten Basic Principles of Catheter Maintenance

1. To preclude leaving the balloon accidentally wedged, do pressure readings in this order: PAW, PA, RA.

2. Always inflate balloon slowly and only to the point that wedge is obtained.

3. Note amount of air needed to wedge balloon with each inflation and compare with amount needed at time of insertion. If it is less, suspect that the catheter may be migrating into a permanent wedge position with baloon deflated. See figure 5.31.

4. NEVER use fluids to inflate the balloon.

5. Ensure against accidental inflation of the balloon with fluids; either keep an empty syringe on the balloon port (no air in the syringe barrel) or disconnect syringe from the balloon port.

6. Never leave the balloon wedged for longer than is absolutely necessary to obtain PAW. One to 2 minutes is the absolute maximum for

most patients, while 15 seconds is the maximum for elderly patients and those with pulmonary hypertension.

7. Do not aspirate the air from an inflated balloon. Instead, simply disconnect the syringe so that the balloon may deflate passively.

8. Avoid drawing routine blood samples and giving vasoactive drugs through the PA or RA ports. The former will lead to premature obstruction of the lumen from fibrin buildup; the latter increases the risk of inadvertent injection of potent vasoactive drugs.

9. Change the dressing over the insertion site at least daily; report signs of inflammation and exudation promptly.

10. When entering an indwelling line for blood sampling or infusion of fluids, maintain strict sterile technique.

B. Common PA Catheter Problems

1. Damped Waveforms (There are many causes; the following are the most common.)

Cause

Air bubbles in the pressure tubing system

Action

Aspirate or purge bubbles from the system.

Cause

Clot in the catheter

Action

Aspirate fluid through the catheter to remove all clots. DO NOT FLUSH FORWARD UNTIL you are *absolutely* certain that there are no clots in any part of the catheter. If normal waveforms do not return after aspirating, the catheter may have to be removed and replaced.

Cause

Kink in the lines

Action

Check the tubing for kinks, including beneath the dressing.

Cause

Overwedged catheter

Action

Pull the catheter out of permanent wedge position (according to hospital policy).

2. Blood in the Pressure Tubing (This happens when the patient's blood pressure exceeds the pressure within the pressure monitoring system.)

Cause

Low bag pressure

Action

Turn most proximal stopcock off *toward* the patient and pump the pressure bag to the proper level; then purge the blood from the line into a syringe to assure that no clots remain before flushing forward. If blood gets into diaphragm, set up a new transducer dome, as waveform may become damped.

Cause

Loose connections or leaks in the pressure monitoring system

Action

Use sterile 4 × 4s to wipe suspect area, observe for leaks, tighten or replace defective fittings.

3. PA Wave Becomes RV

Cause

Displacement of the catheter tip, as seen when the catheter tip recoils from PA to RV

Action

Inflate the balloon while monitoring for PVCs. If the catheter tip does not travel to PA and wedge, have the physician reposition the catheter. After deflating the balloon, the nurse may pull the catheter back to RA if PVCs are frequent.[a]

4. PA Wave Becomes Permanently Wedged

Cause

The catheter tip migrates from PA to permanent wedge position with the balloon deflated (see figure 5.30).

Actions

Be sure that RA is not being monitored instead of PAW and that module is on correct scale; then proceed as follows:

a. Extend the right arm (if insertion site is right brachial), change patient to side-lying position, and ask the patient to cough.

---

[a] If covered by written hospital policy.

b. Withdraw catheter 1 to 2 cm[b] and obtain an x-ray to check catheter tip position.

ALERT REPOSITION THE CATHETER *AS SOON AS POSSIBLE* TO PREVENT POSSIBLE PULMONARY INFARCT

5. RA Wave Becomes RV

Cause

RA lumen migrated to RV (see figure 5.21)

---

[b]MD does this; RN can do if covered by written hospital protocol.

Action

Inflate the balloon and notify MD. Reposition or replace the catheter[c] *as soon as possible* to prevent ventricular tachycardia or fibrillation.

6. Catheter Whip/Fling

Cause

Resonance of fluids in the pressure tubing (figure 5.32)

Action

Keep the pressure tubing as short as possible.

Cause

Turbulent blood flow in the PA causes the catheter to whip around; hence, markedly different pressures and waveforms

---

[c]MD does this; RN can do if covered by written hospital protocol.

Action

Calculate mean pressures (see page xx), or use mechanical damping device.

7. Faulty Measurements

Cause

Each inch the transducer or air zero port is above or below the right atrium will result in a 2 mm Hg error. If the zero port is high, the pressures will be erroneously low; if the zero port is too low, the readings will be high (see figure 3.1).

Action

Level the transducer or zero port with the patient's RA.

C. Dressing Changes

Dressings must be changed daily and prn,[d] using *strict* aseptic technique.

1. Supplies

  a. Transparent or occlusive dressing materials
  b. Sterile gloves
  c. Betadine Swabsticks/Solution
  d. Betadine Ointment
  e. Sterile 4 × 4s

2. Procedure

  a. Carefully remove and discard old dressing (catheter is not always sutured in place).
  b. Pour Betadine Solution into sterile containers.

---

[d]May vary among hospitals.

c. Glove and observe site for swelling, warmth, redness, exudate, or tenderness. Notify physician if any present.

d. Note markings on the catheter to determine position of insertion.

e. Clean site with Betadine Solution and 4 × 4s/Swabsticks using a circular motion, beginning at insertion site and moving away from it in ever-increasing circles. Use a new 4 × 4/Swabstick for each cleansing; cleanse until all exudate is removed.

f. Place Betadine Ointment over insertion and suture sites, and cover with a transparent or occlusive dressing.

1) if a *brachial* catheter, anchor with two pieces of tape twisted in a chevron style; put tape *only* 3/4 of way around arm

2) if a *subclavian* or *jugular* catheter, tape catheter to patient's forehead to minimize tension when patient turns head

g. Do NOT tourniquet limbs with tape.

h. Chart findings.

D. Removing the PA Catheter

This procedure is done by an MD or RN, according to hospital policy.

1. Supplies and Equipment
   a. Sterile gloves
   b. Suture removal set
   c. Sterile 4 × 4s
   d. Betadine Ointment
   e. Dressing material
   f. Defibrillator at the bedside
2. Points to Remember
   a. Be certain the balloon is *deflated* before withdrawing the catheter.
   b. The catheter should withdraw without resistance; if any resistance is encountered, STOP. Pulling against resistance could cause serious damage.
   c. PVCs may occur as the catheter passes through the right ventricle.

d. Bleeding may occur at the insertion site. Apply immediate manual pressure the instant the catheter tip is out. Continue this pressure until the bleeding is checked. (Heparinized patients may require 5 minutes or more of manual pressure.) Apply a pressure dressing.

E. Electrical Safety

Electrical safety is of great importance in all areas of the hospital, and especially so in the critical care setting for patients with Swan-Ganz catheters in place. While your hospital safety manual will contain an electrical safety protocol, below are listed several points the authors choose to emphasize.

1. Patients with PA catheters in place should be in nonelectric beds. If an electric bed is used, disconnect the power cord from the wall outlet.

2. All electrical equipment must be properly grounded and checked periodically to ensure that there is no leakage of current.

3. The thermistor connector on the PA catheter must be capped when not being used for measuring cardiac output. The PA catheter should not be connected to the cardiac output computer during insertion or at any time when cardiac outputs are not being done.

4. Do not make contact with any electrical equipment when handling the PA catheter.

5. Keep the environment dry at all times. This includes bed linens, PA catheter, cardiac output computer, and the monitor cable.

6. Do not operate anything electrical, including the cardiac output computer, when explosive anesthetic agents are present.

3. Procedure

ALERT IF PATIENT HAS A PACEMAKER, THE PA CATHETER MUST BE WITHDRAWN BY AN MD UNDER FLUOROSCOPY, TO AVOID DISPLACEMENT OF THE PACING WIRES.

a. Remove the occlusive dressing from the insertion site.
b. Put on sterile gloves.

c. Remove sutures.

d. With a folded 4 × 4 in one hand, use the other hand to withdraw the catheter. Use the folded 4 × 4 to apply manual pressure.

e. When the bleeding has been controlled, apply Betadine Ointment and dressing. Check frequently for bleeding: q15 min × 4, q30 min × 2, q1 h × 5, and prn.

Appendix 2   Troubleshooting the PA Catheter

When troubleshooting the PA catheter, remove the dressing and inspect the catheter from the module to the insertion site. Check these common causes of malfunction and troubleshoot in this sequence:

1. Electrical modules (tighten all fittings).
2. Transducer and lines (balance and flush transducer).
3. Recorder-amplifier (zero and calibrate accurately).
4. Monitor channels (use correct scale).
5. Stopcocks (turn all in proper direction).
6. Damaged equipment (replace parts suspected to be damaged).

Appendix 3 Maneuvers to Eradicate Line Damping

1. **Determine that the PA catheter is not in the wedge position.** Check that the catheter has not migrated by comparing the present cm mark at the insertion site with the original or previous cm indexing mark.

2. **Withdraw blood samples.** Using a 3 ml syringe, withdraw blood from the PA and RA ports. Air bubbles in these samples may indicate a broken or leaking balloon. Inject 0.5 ml of air through balloon port and redraw blood samples. If air bubbles are present, close balloon port and do not attempt PAW readings.

3. **Hand flush the PA and RA ports.** Use a 10 ml syringe filled with heparinized flush solution to flush the PA and RA ports. *Note:* Never hand flush an arterial catheter.

4. **Inflate balloon and flush catheter.** Partially inflate the balloon and simultaneously flush the PA and RA lines. If the catheter is adhering to the wall of a blood vessel, this procedure may allow it to float free.

Appendix 4   Infection Prevention and Control

The use of intravascular lines for venous access and arterial and/or hemodynamic monitoring increases the risk of nosocomial infection, too often resulting in significant morbidity and mortality. Factors contributing to line sepsis are listed below.

1. Poor technique during insertion.
2. Length of time the lines are left in place (for instance, plastic catheters left in place for more than 3 days are associated with a bacteremia rate as high as 8%).
3. Type of solution being infused (for instance, Hyperol and lipids enhance growth of microorganisms).
4. Age of patient.
5. Disease process, especially when immunosuppression and infection are present.
6. Surgery that requires multiple lines.

Line-associated bacteremia may be suspected under the following conditions:

1. An appropriate microorganism is isolated from the blood.
2. Clinical evidence is found in a patient with a line that has been in place more than 72 hours and no other source of infection is evident.

Action

Remove the line and culture the catheter tip. If more than 15 colonies are isolated, bacteremia is present, and the same organism is isolated from the blood, the catheter is considered the source of sepsis.

Closed System Hemodynamic Monitoring Set-Ups

During the past several years, closed system tubing set-ups for hemodynamic monitoring have come on the market. Theoretically, these systems represent a significant breakthrough in reducing the incidence of nosocomial infection through the hemodynamic monitoring process, since there are not the myriad of connections to contaminate during the initial setting up procedure, or later, when any of the connections would, could, and did come apart.

However, theory notwithstanding, at the time of this writing, studies have not demonstrated the much hoped for significant reduction in line contamination by using the newly designed closed systems, even though we know that the fewer components there are to contaminate, the safer the system should be. Studies available at this time, unfortunately, do not offer conclusive proof of significantly improved patient safety by using the closed systems over the multiple jointed tubing and iced syringe technique. This could well be the result of factors not yet identified or simply poor technique. For this reason, we recommend that you use good aseptic technique with all lines and follow the guidelines listed in tables 1 and 2 of this appendix. Also, please refer to the manufacturers' literature on setting up any of the various closed system pressure tubing systems.

Table 1 Line-related Sepsis: Control Measures[a]

Source	Usual Organism	Control Measures
Catheter related		
Peripheral	Staphylococcus aureus	Handwashing
Arterial	S. epidermidis	Aseptic insertion technique
Central (triple lumen)	Candida	Change lines
		Peripheral q 3 days
		Arterial q 4 days
		Central q 7 days
Infusate related	Klebsiella	Removal of contaminated lots
	Enterobacter	
	Serratia	
	Pseudomonas cepacia/maltophilia	
	Flavobacterium	

| Tubing related | Klebsiella
Enterobacter
Serratia | Remove all possibly contaminated IV solutions, flush solutions, and medications |
| | P. cepacia/maltophilia
Flavobacterium | Change tubing q 3 days
Avoid manipulating stopcocks |

[a]Adapted from Yannelli B, Gurevich I: Infection control in critical care. *Heart Lung*, November 1988, Vol. 17, No. 6, Pt. 1:596–600.

Table 2   CDC Guidelines for the Prevention of Infections Related to Intravascular Pressure Monitoring Systems[a]

Component	Recommendation	Category[b]
Flush solution	Change q 24 hours	1
Chamber dome	Change q 48 hours	2

Tubing and continuous flow device	Change q 48 hours	2
Transducer disinfection between different patients	High level disinfection with chemical agent or sterilize with ethylene oxide	1
Transducer disinfection during prolonged use by a single patient	No recommendation	No recommendation

[a]Adapted from Sawyer Sommers M, Baas L.S., and Beiting A.M. Nosocomial infection related to four methods of hemodynamic monitoring. Heart Lung, January 1987, Vol. 16, No. 1, 13–19.

[b]Category 1, strongly recommended for adoption and strongly supported by well-designed and controlled clinical studies; category 2, moderately recommended for adoption and supported by highly suggestive clinical studies.

Appendix 5   Cardiac Therapy Indicated by Subsets of Hemodynamic Parameters[a]

Subset: Normal Hemodynamics

HR	nml[b]
BP	nml
CO	nml
PAW	nml

Therapy: 1. Decrease cardiac workload and O_2 consumption.
2. Give sedation, calcium blockers, beta blockers.

Subset: Decreased LV Compliance

HR	nml

---

[a]May vary according to patient's clinical status, physician's preference, and/or hospital protocol.
[b]nml = normal; inc = increased; dec = decreased.

BP	nml
CO	nml
PAW	inc[b]

Therapy: 1. Compensate for decreased LV compliance.
2. Give diuretics.

Subset: Pulmonary Edema

HR	inc
BP	inc
CO	inc
PAW	inc

Therapy: 1. Treat for pulmonary edema.
2. Reduce preload (e.g., nitrates) and afterload (e.g., diuretics).

Subset: Hyperdynamic State

HR	nml-inc

APPENDIX 5: Cardiac Therapy Indicated by Subsets of Hemodynamic Parameters   177

BP   inc
CO   inc
PAW   inc

Therapy: 1. Differentiate hyperdynamic state from pulmonary edema by etiology.
2. Treat the cause.

Subset: Hypovolemia

HR   inc
BP   nml-dec[b]
CO   nml-dec
PAW   dec

Therapy: 1. Treat for hypovolemia.
2. Replace fluids as needed.

Subset: Shock Syndrome

HR   inc

BP	dec
CO	dec
PAW	dec

Therapy: 1. Treat for specific shock syndrome (hypovolemic, anaphylactic, septic).

2. Increase volume and give vasopressors.

Subset: Cardiogenic Shock

HR	inc
BP	dec
CO	dec
PAW	inc

Therapy: 1. Treat for cardiogenic shock.

2. Give vasopressors; reduce afterload (e.g., with nitroprusside, intraaortic balloon counter pulsation).

APPENDIX 5: Cardiac Therapy Indicated by Subsets of Hemodynamic Parameters   179

Appendix 6   Definitions

Afterload

The resistance (or difficulty) a ventricle encounters while expelling its content. For the left ventricle, afterload comprises the resistance associated with the aortic valve apparatus, the diastolic aortic pressure, the compliance of the aorta, and the peripheral vascular resistance. For clinical purposes, in the presence of normal aortic valve function, the latter is the most important factor.

Afterload Reduction

Therapy aimed at reducing the resistance to left ventricular ejection. Ventricular volume remains the same or is decreased, but cardiac output increases. This is accomplished with drugs that decrease peripheral vascular resistance or intraaortic balloon counterpulsation, which reduces intraaortic pressure during systole (deflation). Systolic unloading increases the stroke volume at the same end-diastolic fiber length. Heart size is decreased by more complete emptying, and this, in turn, decreases myocardial oxygen demand and cardiac work.

Body Surface Area (BSA)

Body size, stated in meters squared (m^2), calculated by multiplying height and weight and a constant representing a factor that converts units of inches and pounds into units of area. See formula, Appendix 8.

Cardiac Index (CI)

The volume of cardiac output per square meter of body surface area per minute. This eliminates differences of weight and body size and standardizes cardiac output. See formula, Appendix 8.

Cardiac Output (CO)

The volume of blood ejected by the left ventricle in 1 minute. See formula, Appendix 8.

Catheter Whip/Fling

Artifactual variation on a pressure tracing caused by movement of the tip or shaft of the PA catheter within the pulmonary artery.

Compliance

Expandability, elasticity, or distensibility of the myocardial wall. High compliance = easily stretched myocardial fibers/wall. Low compliance = little distensibility = stiff myocardial fibers/wall.

Contractility

The ability of the heart muscle to change its force of contraction, independent of preload or afterload. This is accomplished by release of norepinephrine, intracellular calcium stores, and circulating catecholamines. Myocardial contractility can be affected by inotropic agent, pharmacologic depressants, physiologic depressants (e.g., hypoxia, hypercapnia, acidosis), and loss of ventricular mass.

Damping

Decreased amplitude of pressure tracings, because of factors that depress true pressure transmission through a catheter, a transducer dome, or stopcock.

Ejection Fraction

The proportion of the blood volume in the ventricle at the end of diastole that is ejected during systole. Normal value at rest is 55% to 65%; during exercise, 60% to 80%.

End-Expiratory Pressure

The pressure readings taken at the end of one expiration and before the next inspiration. This is the most accurate reading for PA and PAW, since intrathoracic pressures are most stable and reproducible at this time.

Left Ventricular Diastolic Pressure (LVDP)

The pressure in the left ventricle at the end of diastole, just before contraction. This provides a rough estimate of the volume of the left ventricle and is the earliest indicator of alteration of filling and functioning of the left ventricle.

Mean Arterial Pressure (MAP)

The average pressure in the peripheral arterial system during the entire cardiac cycle. With normal heart rate, it is closer to the diastolic pressure than the systolic, since diastole lasts for two-thirds of the cardiac cycle. As the heart rate increases, MAP may be closer to the systolic pressure, as ventricular filling time decreases. See formula, Appendix 8.

Mixed Venous Blood

Blood that has circulated through the system and is lower in O_2 and higher in CO_2, compared with arterial blood. The value is the pooled average of the blood from organs with differing metabolic needs. A mixed venous blood sample is drawn from the pulmonary artery. See Appendix 4.

Oxygen Concentration: Arterial-Venous Difference

The difference in oxygen content between arterial and venous blood. If cardiac output is low, increased extraction of oxygen by the tissues will reduce the venous blood saturation percentage and widen the AV difference. Normal range is 3.0 to 5.5 volumes/percent of saturation.

Oxygen Content

The amount of oxygen present in the blood. It is calculated by measuring oxyhemoglobin and multiplying by the theoretical oxygen-carrying capacity of the blood (1.34 ml of O_2/gm of hemoglobin).

Preload

The stretch that develops in the muscle fibers of the ventricular wall at the end of diastole. This stretch is influenced by circulating volume, intra- or extrathoracic distribution of circulating volume, and atrial contraction.

Preload Reduction

Therapy aimed at reducing end-diastolic stretch. It is accomplished with drugs that reduce circulating volume, such as diuretics, or cause peripheral venous dilation and decreased venous return.

Pulmonary Artery Wedge Pressure (PAW)

When the balloon of the PA catheter is inflated, it floats into and occludes a small branch of the pulmonary artery, and the pressure of the pulmonary capillary bed (LA/LVDP) is measured.

Pulmonary Hypertension

Pulmonary artery pressure above accepted limits of normal (35/15 mm Hg). PAW will usually be normal.

Pulmonary Vascular Resistance (PVR)

Resistance offered to right ventricular ejection by the pulmonary vascular bed. It is directly proportional to the pressure drop across the pulmonary bed and inversely proportional to the rate of blood flow. PVR is calculated by measuring the inflow pressure (mean pulmonary artery pressure), less the outflow pressure (mean pulmonary artery wedge pressure), and dividing by cardiac output. See formula, Appendix 8.

Starling's Law

The more that the myocardial fibers are stretched during diastole, the more they will shorten (contract) during systole, and the greater the force of contraction.

Stroke Volume (SV)

The amount of blood ejected by the left ventricle per beat. This is determined by preload, afterload, and contractility. See formula, Appendix 8.

Stroke Volume Index

A measurement that standardizes stroke volume to body size. See formula, Appendix 8.

Stroke Work

A measurement of the amount of ventricular work per heart beat. It is calculated by taking mean arterial pressure, less the ventricular diastolic pressure, and multiplying by stroke volume and a conversion factor that changes pressure to work. See formula, Appendix 8.

Stroke Work Index

A method that standardizes stroke work to body size. See formula, Appendix 8.

Systemic Vascular Resistance (SVR)

Resistance to outflow from aorta and great vessels by the systemic vascular bed. It is directly proportional to the pressure drop across the systemic bed and inversely proportional to cardiac output. SVR is calculated by measuring the outflow pressure (mean arterial pressure), less the inflow pressure (mean right atrial pressure), and dividing by cardiac output. See formula, Appendix 8.

Transducer

A device that converts the mechanical pressures transmitted by the fluid column in the pressure tubing into electrical signals that can be read on an oscilloscope.

Appendix 7 Commonly Used Vasoactive Drugs and Nomograms[a]

Dobutamine HCl (Dobutrex)

Uses
1. Treat cardiogenic shock.
2. Short-term treatment of decompensation.

Dosage
1. Commonly, 2.5-10 µg/kg/min IV drip.
2. Occasionally, doses to 40 µg/kg/min.

Adverse
1. Increased heart rate, PVCs, increased systolic blood pressure.
2. Increased AV conduction (for patients with atrial fib, digitalize prior to starting Dobutrex).
3. Nausea, headache, dyspnea, angina, palpitations.

---

[a]Courtesy of Meg Fears, RN, MS, Loma Linda Hospice, Loma Linda, California.

Dobutamine

250 mg Dobutamine / 250 cc D5W

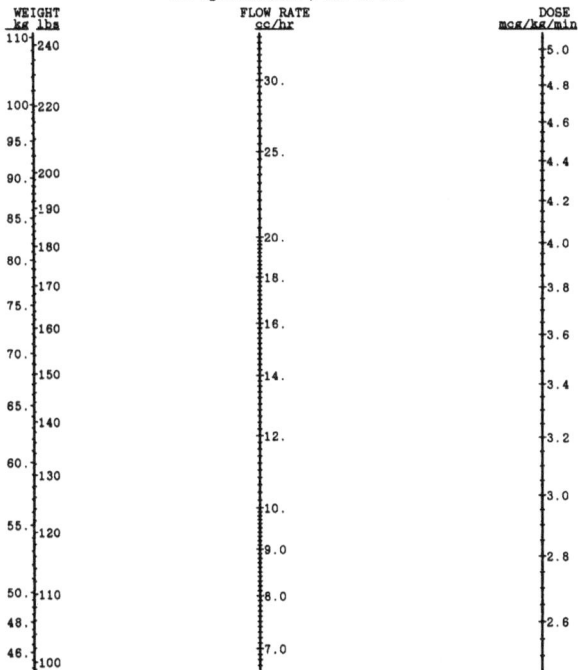

```
WEIGHT              FLOW RATE                    DOSE
kg  lbs               cc/hr                   mcg/kg/min

110┬240                                         ┬5.0
   ┤                  ┬30.                       ┤
100┼220               ┤                          ┤4.8
95.┤                  ┤                          ┤4.6
   ┤                  ┼25.                        ┤
90.┼200               ┤                          ┤4.4
85.┼190               ┤                          ┤4.2
   ┤                  ┤                          ┤
80.┼180               ┼20.                       ┤4.0
   ┼170               ┼18.                       ┤3.8
75.┤                  ┤                          ┤
   ┼160               ┼16.                       ┤3.6
70.┤                  ┤                          ┤
   ┼150               ┼14.                       ┤3.4
65.┤                  ┤                          ┤
   ┼140               ┼12.                       ┤3.2
60.┤                  ┤                          ┤
   ┼130               ┤                          ┤3.0
   ┤                  ┼10.                       ┤
55.┼120               ┼9.0                       ┤2.8
   ┤                  ┤                          ┤
50.┼110               ┼8.0                       ┤2.6
48.┤                  ┤                          ┤
46.┼100               ┼7.0
```

Example: 3 mcg/kg/min for a 70 kg patient requires 12.6 cc/hr

Note: At 60 drops per cc, 1 cc/hr <----> 1 drop/min
       At 10 drops per cc, 1 cc/hr ----> 1/6 drop/min,
                           1 drop/min ----> 6 cc/hr

APPENDIX 7: Commonly Used Vasoactive Drugs and Nomograms

Intropin (Dopamine)

Uses
1. Treatment of choice for cardiogenic shock.
2. Treat decompensation.
3. Increase renal perfusion.

Dosage
1. Titrate 2-50 µg/kg/min for cardiogenic shock.
2. Titrate 2-5 µg/kg/min for renal perfusion.

Adverse
1. Dysrhythmias.
2. Nausea, vomiting, dyspnea, headache.
3. Hypertension, vasoconstriction.

Note: pH incompatibility with sodium bicarbonate. Do not mix Dopamine with $NaHCO_3$.

Dopamine
400 mg Dopamine / 250 cc D5W

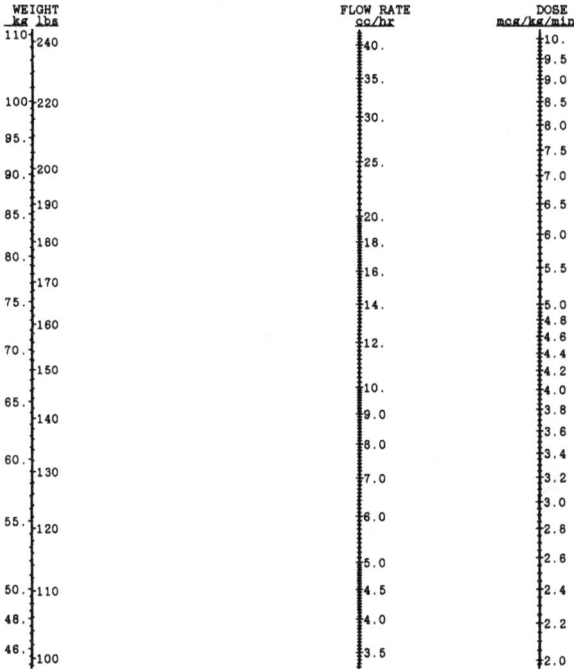

```
WEIGHT              FLOW RATE           DOSE
 kg  lbs              cc/hr           mcg/kg/min
110                    40.               10.
     240                                  9.5
                       35.                9.0
100  220                                  8.5
                       30.                8.0
 95.                                      7.5
                       25.
 90.  200                                 7.0
 85.  190                                 6.5
                       20.
 80.  180              18.                6.0
                                          5.5
      170              16.
 75.                   14.                5.0
      160                                 4.8
                       12.                4.6
 70.                                      4.4
      150                                 4.2
                       10.                4.0
 65.                    9.0               3.8
      140
                        8.0               3.6
 60.                                      3.4
      130               7.0               3.2
                                          3.0
 55.  120               6.0               2.8
                        5.0               2.6
 50.  110               4.5               2.4
 48.                    4.0               2.2
 46.  100               3.5               2.0
```

Example: 5   mcg/kg/min for a 84 kg patient requires 15.7 cc/hr
Note: At 60 drops per cc, 1 cc/hr <----> 1 drop/min
       At 10 drops per cc, 1 cc/hr ----> 1/6 drop/min,
                           1 drop/min ----> 6 cc/hr

Isoproteronol (Isuprel)

Uses
1. Increase pacemaker automaticity and AV conduction.
2. Treat cardiogenic shock.
3. Bronchodilation.

Dosage
1. IV: titrate 0.5-5 µg/kg/min.
2. IC: 0.02 mg direct push over 1-2 minutes.

Adverse
1. SVT, PVCs, V-tach, V-fib.
2. Hypotension from vasodilation.
3. Headache, flushing, angina, nausea, tremor, vertigo, weakness, sweating.

Nitroglycerin

Uses
1. Prophylaxis and treatment of angina, both acute and chronic.
2. Produce controlled hypotension during surgery.

3. Treat CHF associated with MI and ischemic episodes (preload reduction).

Dosage 1. Topical: 2% Ungt: start with 1/2 inch and increase until desired effect is reached. Usual topical dose is 1-2 inches TID.
2. Sublingual: 0.2-0.6 mg for acute angina. May repeat every 5 minutes for 3 doses.
3. Oral: 1 sustained release capsule every 8-12 hours.
4. IV: start at 5 μg/min and titrate up every 3-5 minutes until desired effect is reached.

Adverse 1. Hypotension (especially orthostatic), flushing, tachycardia, syncope.
2. Headache, vertigo, weakness.
3. Nausea, vomiting.

APPENDIX 7: Commonly Used Vasoactive Drugs and Nomograms

Nitroglycerine

50 mg Nitroglycerine / 250 cc D5W

WEIGHT kg lbs	FLOW RATE cc/hr	DOSE mcg/kg/min
110 — 240	800	
		24.
100 — 220	700	
95.	600	22.
90. — 200		20.
85. — 190	500	19.
80. — 180	450	18.
75. — 170	400	17.
	350	16.
70. — 160		
— 150	300	15.
65. — 140		14.
60.	250	13.
— 130		
55. — 120	200	12.
	180	
50. — 110	160	11.
48.		
46. — 100	140	10.

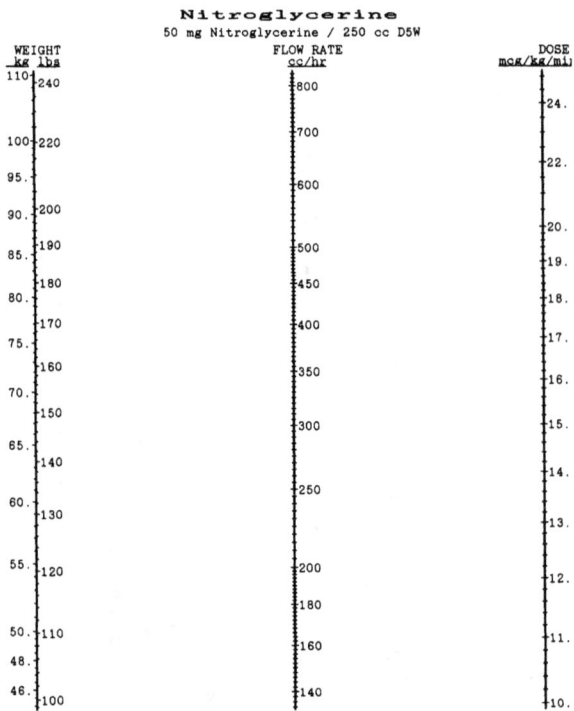

Example: 20 mcg/kg/min for a 65 kg patient requires 390 cc/hr
Note: At 60 drops per cc, 1 cc/hr <----> 1 drop/min
        At 10 drops per cc, 1 cc/hr ----> 1/6 drop/min,
                            1 drop/min ----> 6 cc/hr

Nitroprusside Sodium (Nipride)

Uses
1. Immediate treatment of hypertensive crisis.
2. Produce controlled hypotension during surgery to minimize blood loss.
3. Treat cardiogenic shock (preload and afterload reduction).

Dosage
1. Titrate (not to exceed 10 μg/kg/min).

Adverse
1. Sudden, severe hypotension.
2. Chest and abdominal pain.
3. Neurologic disturbances.
4. Nausea, vomiting.

Nitroprusside

50 mg Nitroprusside / 250 cc D5W

WEIGHT kg lbs	FLOW RATE cc/hr	DOSE mcg/kg/min
110 — 240		10. 9.5 9.0
	300	8.5 8.0
	250	7.5
100 — 220		7.0
	200	6.5
95. —	180	6.0
	160	5.5
90. — 200	140	5.0
85. — 190	120	4.8 4.6 4.4 4.2 4.0
	100	3.8
80. — 180	90.	3.6 3.4
	80.	3.2
75. — 170	70.	3.0
	60.	2.8
		2.6
75. — 160	50.	2.4
70. —	45.	2.2
	40.	2.0 1.9
150	35.	1.8 1.7
65. — 140	30.	1.6 1.5
	25.	1.4
60. — 130		1.3 1.2
	20.	1.1
	18.	
55. — 120	16.	1.0 .95 .90
	14.	.85 .80
	12.	.75
50. — 110	10.	.70
48. —	9.0	.65
	8.0	.60
46. — 100	7.0	.55 .50

Example: 8   mcg/kg/min for a   55   kg patient requires   132   cc/hr
Note: At 60 drops per cc, 1 cc/hr <----> 1 drop/min
       At 10 drops per cc, 1 cc/hr ----> 1/6 drop/min,
                           1 drop/min ----> 6 cc/hr

Norephinephrine (Levophed)

Uses
1. Treat cardiogenic shock.
2. Treat other forms of hypotension.

Dosage
1. 2-4 µg/min IV.
2. Titrate solution for desired effect.

Adverse
1. Severe hypertension.
2. Tissue sloughing from infiltration (use a central line if one is available).
3. Many and varied dysrhythmias.
4. Anxiety, headache.

Verapamil (Calan, Isoptin)

Uses
1. Manage stable and chronic angina.
2. Manage Prinzmetal's or variant (vasospastic) angina.

Dosage 1. Oral: 80 mg 3-4 times a day. Maintenance dose may be as high as 480 mg/day.
2. IV: 5-10 mg slow IVP or IVPB (with BP and EKG monitoring). Repeat in 30 minutes PRN.

Adverse 1. Bradycardia, transient hypotension, CHF, AV block, asystole.
2. Vertigo, headache, fatigue.
3. Nausea, constipation, elevated liver function tests.

Appendix 8 Formulas

A. Body Surface Area (BSA)

$BSA = weight^{0.425} \times height^{0.725} \times 71.84$

W = weight (in kg)
H = height (in cm)
71.84 = conversion factor (inches and pounds to area) OR use Du-
Bois Body Surface Chart, Appendix 11

B. Cardiac Output (CO)

$CO = SV \times HR$

SV = stroke volume
HR = heart rate
Normal range = 4-8 liters/min/m^2

C. Cardiac Index (CI)

CI = CO ÷ BSA

CO = cardiac output
BSA = body surface area

Normal range = 3.2-5.2 liters/min/m^2

D. Mean Arterial Pressure (MAP)[a]

MAP = (S + 2D) ÷ 3

S = systolic pressure
D = diastolic pressure

Normal range = 80-100 mm Hg

E. Pulmonary Vascular Resistance (PVR)

PVR = mean PA − PAW(80) ÷ CO

---

[a]Same formula is used to calculate mean PA pressure. Normal range mean PA = 9-19 mm Hg.

PA   = pulmonary artery
PAW = pulmonary artery wedge
CO   = cardiac output

Normal value = 20-120 dyne/sec/cm^{-5}

F. Stroke Volume (SV)

SV = CO(1000) ÷ HR

CO = cardiac output
HR = heart rate

Normal range = 60-100 ml/beat

G. Stroke Volume Index (SVI)

SVI = CI(1000) ÷ HR

CI = cardiac index
HR = heart rate

Normal range = 33-47 ml/beat/m^2

H. Stroke Work (SW)

SW = (MAP − VED) × SV × 0.0144

MAP = mean arterial pressure
VED = ventricular end-diastolic pressure
SV = stroke volume
0.0144 = conversion factor (pressure to work)

Normal range = 45-85 ml/beat/m^2

I. Stroke Work Index (SWI)

SWI = (MAP − PAW) × SV × 0.0144 ÷ BSA

MAP = mean arterial pressure
PAW = pulmonary artery wedge
SV = stroke volume
0.0144 = conversion factor (pressure to work)
BSA = body surface area

Normal range = 40-80 gm/beat/m^2

J. Systemic Vascular Resistance (SVR)

SVR = (MAP − MRAP)(80) ÷ CO

$\quad$ *MAP = mean arterial pressure*
$\quad$ *MRAP = mean right atrial pressure*
$\quad$ *CO = cardiac output*

Normal value = 800-1200 dyne/sec/cm^{-5}

K. Converting mg/ml to μ/ml:

Multiply mg/ml by 1,000 and divide by volume.
Example: 400 mg/250 ml = 400,000 μg/250 ml = 1,600 μg/ ml.

L. Converting μg/kg/min:

Concentration in μg/kg × 60 × μgtts/min.
Example: 1,600 μg/100 kg × 60 × 15 μgtts/min = 4 μg/kg/min.

Appendix 9 Blood Gases

Arterial Blood Gases (ABGs): Normal Values

$$pH = 7.35\text{-}7.45$$
$$pCO_2 = 35\text{-}45$$
$$pO_2 = 85+$$
$$O_2 \text{ sat.} = 94\%+$$

Mixed Venous Blood Gases: Normal Values

$$pH = 7.37\text{-}7.42$$
$$pCO_2 = 40\text{-}46$$
$$pO_2 = 36+$$
$$O_2 \text{ sat.} = 70\%+$$

In order to draw a mixed venous sample from the distal port, the PA catheter must be in a central portion of the pulmonary artery bed. If it is in a peripheral branch, the sampling will be inaccurate.

Draw mixed venous samples slowly (approximately 1 ml/min for a 3 ml sample) to avoid aspirating oxygenated capillary blood, thus giving a false increased pO_2 of mixed venous sample. Leave balloon *deflated*; flush catheter with heparinized solution.

Appendix 10   Hemodynamic Parameters

	Average (mg Hg)	Range (mg Hg)
Right atrium		
Mean	2.8	2–6
A wave (relative)	5.6	2.5–7
C wave (relative)	3.8	1.5–6
V wave (relative)	4.6	2–7.5
Right ventricle		
Peak systolic	25	17–32
End-diastolic	2–6	1–7
Pulmonary artery		
Mean	15	9–19
Peak systolic	25	17–32
End-diastolic	8–12	4–13
PAW		
Mean		8–12

A wave (relative)	5.6	2.5–7
C wave (relative)	3.8	1.5–6
V wave (relative)	4.6	2–7.5
Cardiac output		4–8 liters/min/m²
Cardiac index		3.2–5.2 liters/min/m²
Ejection fraction		55%–65%
Mean arterial pressure		80–100 mm Hg
Mean pulmonary artery pressure		9–19 mm Hg
Pulmonary vascular resistance		20–120 dyne/sec/cm^{-5}
Oxygen content (A/V difference)		3.5–5.5 volume percent
Stroke volume		60–100 ml/beat
Stroke volume index		33–47 ml/beat/m²
Stroke work		45–85 ml/beat/m²
Stroke work index		40–80 gm/beat/m²
Systemic vascular resistance		800–1200 dyne/sec/cm^{-5}

Appendix 11   BSA Chart

To find body surface area of a patient, locate the height in inches (or centimeters) on Scale I and the weight in pounds (or kilograms) on Scale II and place a straight edge (ruler) between these two points which will intersect Scale III at the patient's surface area.[a]

---

[a]From Eugene F. DuBois, *Basal Metabolism in Health and Disease*. Philadelphia: Lea and Febiger, 1936. Copyright 1920 by W. M. Boothby and R. B. Sandiford.

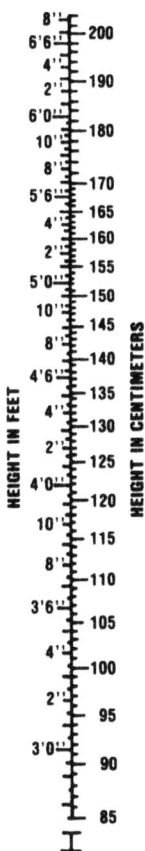

HEIGHT IN FEET

HEIGHT IN CENTIMETERS

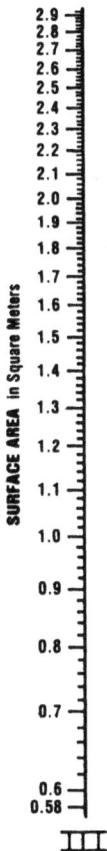

SURFACE AREA in Square Meters

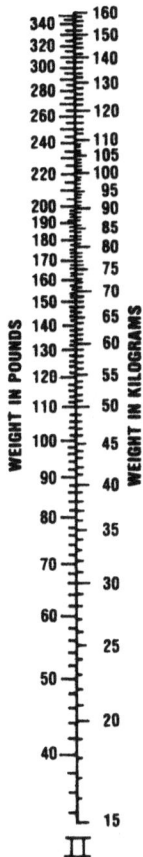

WEIGHT IN POUNDS

WEIGHT IN KILOGRAMS

APPENDIX 11: BSA Chart 211

Appendix 12   Abbreviations

CI	cardiac index	PAW	pulmonary artery wedge
CO	cardiac output	$\overline{PAW}$	mean pulmonary artery wedge
CVP	central venous pressure	PVR	pulmonary vascular resistance
LAP	left atrial pressure	RA	right atrium
LVP	left ventricular pressure	RV	right ventricle
LVDP	left ventricular diastolic pressure	RVDP	right ventricular diastolic pressure
MAP	mean arterial pressure	SV	stroke volume
PA	pulmonary artery	SVI	stroke volume index
$\overline{PA}$	mean pulmonary artery	SVR	systemic vascular resistance
PAD	pulmonary artery diastolic pressure	SW	stroke work
PAS	pulmonary artery systolic pressure	SWI	stroke work index

Bibliography

Andreoli, V., Zipes, D., Wallace, A., Kinney, M., and Fowkes, V. *Comprehensive Cardiac Care*, ed 6. St. Louis: Mosby, 1987.

Bodai, B., and Holcroft, J. Use of the Pulmonary Arterial Catheter in the Critically Ill Patient. *Heart & Lung*, September–October 1982: 406–415.

Bookbinder, N., and Ganz, W. Hemodynamic monitoring: invasive techniques. *Anesthesiology*, August 1976:146–155.

Brantigan, C. Hemodynamic monitoring: interpreting values. *Am. J. Nurs.*, January 1982:86-89.

Centers for Disease Control. Guidelines for prevention of infections related to intravascular pressure-monitoring systems. Atlanta: *Infection Control 3*, 1982:68.

Daily, E., and Schroeder, J. *Hemodynamic Waveforms, Exercises in Identification and Analysis*. St. Louis: Mosby, 1983.

Forrester, J., Chatterjee, K., and Swan, H. Hemodynamic monitoring in patients with acute myocardial infarction. *JAMA*, October 1973:60-61.

Gregersen, R. A., Underhill, S. L., Detter, J. C., Schmer, G., and Lax, K. Accurate coagulation studies from heparinized radial artery catheters. *Heart & Lung*, November 1987, Vol. 16, No. 6:686-692.

Hook, M. L., Reuling, J., Luettgen, M. L., O'Brien Norris, S., Elsesser, C. C., and Leonard, M. K. Comparison of the patency of arterial lines maintained with heparinized and nonheparinized infusions. *Heart & Lung*, November 1987, Vol. 16, No. 6:693-698.

Lowe, J., and Fears, M. Nomograms shortcuts to accuracy. *Focus on Critical Care*, June 1986, Vol. 13, No. 3:36-40.

Pattillo, M., and Knox, T. L. Dispute in the intensive care unit; should blood cultures be drawn from arterial lines? *Focus on Critical Care*, October 1987, Vol. 14, No. 5:76–79.

Rakowlski Reinhardt, A. C., Tonneson, A. S., Bracey, A., and Crabtree Goodnough, S. K. Minimum discard volume from arterial catheters to obtain coagulation studies free of heparin effect. *Heart & Lung*, November 1987, Vol. 16, No. 6:699-705.

Sawyer Sommers, M., Baas, L. S., and Beiting, A. M. Nosocomial infections related to four methods of hemodynamic monitoring. *Heart & Lung*, January 1987, Vol. 16, No. 1:13-19.

Truter Von Rueden, K. The effect of hemodynamic monitoring system flush solution on the fluid status of cardiac surgery patients. *Focus on Critical Care*, April 1985, Vol. 12, No. 4:20-23.

Weyant, H. Utilization of an intravenous drug guide. *Focus on Critical Care*, April 1984, Vol. 11, No. 2:58-62.

Yannelli, B. and Gurevich, I. Infection control in critical care. *Heart & Lung*, November 1988, Vol. 17, No. 6, Pt. 1:596-600.

Yonkman, C. A., and Hill Hamory, B. Sterility and efficiency of two methods of cardiac output determination: closed loop and capped syringe methods. *Heart & Lung*, March 1988, Vol. 17, No. 2:121-127.

BANK NOTES

BANK NOTES

BAND NOTES

BANK NOTES

BANK
NOTES

BANK NOTES

BANK NOTES

www.ingramcontent.com/pod-product-compliance
Lightning Source LLC
Chambersburg PA
CBHW060404220326
41598CB00023B/3012